Singh-Mall

Step by Step

Ultrasound
in Obstetrics

System requirement:
- **Windows XP or above**
- **Power DVD player (Software)**
- **Windows Media Player version 10.0 or above**
- **Quick time player version 6.5 or above**

Accompanying CD Rom is playable only in Computer and not in CD player.

Kindly wait for few seconds for CD to autorun. If it does not autorun then please do the following:
- Click on my computer
- Click the **drive labelled JAYPEE** and after opening the drive, kindly double click the file **Jaypee**

Singh-Malhotra Series

Step by Step®

Ultrasound in Obstetrics

2nd Edition

Kuldeep Singh MBBS FAUI FICMCH FICMU
Consultant Ultrasonologist
Special Interest in Obstetric Sonology
in Detailed Anomaly Scanning and
Color Doppler for Management and Gynecological Scanning
**Conducts FOGSI recognised ultrasound training courses in
Obstetrics, Gynecology and Infertility
(Basics, Color Doppler, 3D & 4D)**
Dr Kuldeep's Ultrasound and Color Doppler Clinic
D-80, East of Kailash, New Delhi 110065 (India)
Phones: 011-26441720, 26233342   Mobile: 98111 96613
singhdrkuldeep@rediffmail.com

Narendra Malhotra MD FICOG FICMCH
Consultant and Director
Malhotra Nursing and Maternity Home (P) Ltd., Agra
Apollo Pankaj Hospital (P) Ltd., Agra (India)
President, Federation of Obstetric and Gynaecological
Societies of India—2008
Phones: 0562-2260275, 2260276, 2260277   Mobile: 9837033335
mnmhagra@gmail.com
www.mnmhagra.com, www.mttbc.com
www.narendramalhotra.net

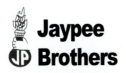

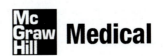

© 2010, Jaypee Brothers Medical Publishers
First published in India in 2008 by

Jaypee Brothers Medical Publishers (P) Ltd.

Corporate Office
4838/24 Ansari Road, Daryaganj, **New Delhi** - 110002, India,
+91-11-43574357

Registered Office
B-3 EMCA House, 23/23B Ansari Road, Daryaganj,
New Delhi 110 002, India
Phones: +91-11-23272143, +91-11-23272703, +91-11-23282021,
+91-11-23245672, Rel: +91-11-32558559 Fax: +91-11-23276490,
+91-11-23245683
e-mail: jaypee@jaypeebrothers.com,
Website: www.jaypeebrothers.com

First published in USA by The McGraw-Hill Companies, 2 Penn Plaza, New York, NY
10121. Exclusively worldwide distributor except South Asia (India, Nepal, Sri Lanka,
Bhutan, Pakistan, Bangladesh, Malaysia).

Set ISBN 978-0-07-166733-3 • MHID 0-07-166733-4
Book PN 9780071667340 • 0071667342
DVD PN 9780071667357 • 0071667350

Preface to the Second Edition

Today ultrasound is the mainstay investigation in all fields of medicine. The widespread use of ultrasound has brought this wonderful technology to the consulting rooms of the practising gynecologists. It is now impossible to even conceive a modern obstetric care unit without ultrasound and it is impossible to practise infertility and gynecology without a transvaginal probe which has added the dimension of imaging with palpation.

Can you even think of a pregnant lady without an ultrasound scan even once: meticulous dating scan, nuchal translucency scan, anomaly scan and biometry scan accompanied with color Doppler help us in managing the pregnancy better and to reduce perinatal morbidity and mortality. It is our pleasure to present to you all the second edition of this book. Your response to the first edition and the feedback from Prof Stuart Campbell has prompted us to improve.

Many more pictures of anomalies especially chromosomal abnormalities have been added to make the reader well-versed with newer markers.

The law in India mandates that each machine and the sonologist be licensed to practise ultrasound under the PCPNDT Act for which training and updating is required.

There are numerous textbooks and reference books on ultrasound but our aim to bring out this handy series of Step by Step Ultrasound in Obstetrics is to simplify the indications, steps and the interpretations of this wonderful technology.

We hope the readers will be benefited by this book.

Kuldeep Singh
Narendra Malhotra

Preface to the First Edition

Today ultrasound is the mainstay investigation in all fields of medicine. The widespread use of ultrasound has brought this wonderful technology to the consulting rooms of the practising gynecologists. It is now impossible to even conceive a modern obstetric care unit without ultrasound and it is impossible to practise infertility and gynecology without a transvaginal probe which has added the dimension of imaging with palpation.

The law in India mandates that each machine and the sonologist be licensed to practise ultrasound under the PNDT Act for which training and updating is required.

There are numerous textbooks and reference books on ultrasound but our aim to bring out this handy series of Step by Step Ultrasound in Obstetrics is to simplify the indications, steps and the interpretations of this wonderful technology.

We hope the readers will be benefited by this book.

Kuldeep Singh
Narendra Malhotra

Acknowledgements

Thanks to our parents, elders, teachers, siblings, daughters, sons and friends for their help in the mamoth project of the 6 step by step books on ultrasound over the years. We have enjoyed writing this series and it is heartening to note that the series is well accepted world over and even translated in Chinese and Spanish languages. This has given us more strength to write the second edition of all the books of the series.

Our sincere thanks to Prof Stuart Campbell and to Prof Asim Kurjak, Sanja Kupesic, Dr Pratap Kumar, Dr PK Shah, Dr Ambrish Dalal, Dr Ashok Khurana and Dr S Suresh and many many others who taught us small tricks of the trade at each step of our life.

Thanks to Jaideep and Nishu for bearing our odd timings and for the support.

Our children Neharika, Keshav, Jaanvi and Ramanjeet, God bless you.

Thanks to Shri JP Vij and the team at M/s Jaypee Brothers Medical Publishers (Pvt) Ltd., for bringing out this wonderful collection.

Contents

Introduction

1.1 FILLING UP OF FORMS

Maintain a form for further follow-up in your clinic. One never knows when the information is required.

The routine information required in these forms is:

a. Name
b. Age
c. Address
d. Telephone number
e. Referred by
f. PNDT Act Form 'F' as required by Government of India Law
g. Undertaking by patient and doctor for obstetric ultrasound with Form 'F'.

1.2 RELEVANT HISTORY

Always spend few minutes with your patient to take the details of the history. Gives confidence to the patient and you get your perspective of what all to expect.

The history to be taken routinely is:

a. Previous obstetric history consisting of details of any abortions (spontaneous or missed), any second or third trimester losses (possible reasons), any previous deliveries (vaginal or cesarean). Try and look into the previous records which can throw any light.

b. Any symptoms in this pregnancy.
c. Any ultrasound done so far in this pregnancy. Check the records carefully.
d. Last menstrual period and regularity of menstrual cycles.
e. Any tests done and their reports.
f. Referring doctors requissition slip (This is now a legal requirement with Form 'F').

1.3 PREPARATION AND POSITIONING OF PATIENT

1. In scans upto 15 weeks a full bladder is required, unless transvaginal. It is preferable to examine upto 12 weeks by a transvaginal scan.
2. Between 15 and 22 weeks holding urine for one hour is sufficient.
3. After 22 weeks no preparation is required. A full bladder for assessment of the cervix and lower segment assessment can be asked for when required.
4. The patient need not be fasting unless and until an upper abdomen scan is also asked for.
5. The patient is almost always scanned supine with plenty of jelly on the abdomen. In certain cases scanning in the lateral position (if patient is uncomfortable lying supine or fetus moves when lying in a lateral position) or with the patient standing (for functional assessment of cervix) is required.
6. Whenever, a transvaginal scan is asked for the bladder must be emptied immediately before the examination. It should be performed with the same respect for privacy and gentleness, as is with the placement of a speculum. Scanning is performed with the patient supine and with her thighs abducted and knees flexed.

Elevation of the buttock may be necessary. The probe should be covered with a condom or sheath containing a small amount of gel. Additional gel should be placed on the outside of sheathed tip. The probe is inserted by a gentle push posteriorly towards the rectum while the patient relaxes. Four types of probe movements are required:

   i. Pushing and pulling
  ii. Rotation
 iii. "Rocking" or upwards and downwards
 iv. Side to side or "Panning".

After removal of the transvaginal probe, the sheath is removed and the coupling gel is wiped off with a damp towel. The TV probe may be disinfected by Cidex.

1.4 MACHINE AND TRANSDUCERS

1. For a transabdominal scan, a 3.5 to 5.0 MHz transducer and for a transvaginal scan, a 5.0 to 8.0 MHz transducer is used.

2. Basic controls of every machine are more or less the same. The placement of knobs is different for all machines. Check for the manual of your machine or somebody from the company can always come and explain you.

    The routine knobology is:

  a. Patient name and entry of last menstrual period after you select the obstetric mode
  b. Freeze
  c. B, B+B, B+M or only M mode
  d. Depth and focus
  e. Overall gain
  f. Time gain (TGC)

   g. Comments on screen
   h. Measurement (Set and select) for linear, area and volume
   i. Track ball or screen or joy stick to move the cursor
   j. Color flow map, Power Doppler, Doppler and 3D and 4D.
   k. After freezing the images these can be stored and a print taken on a camera, thermal printer or from a computer.

1.5 REPORTING

Maximum possible information to be given in the report to the patient.

Routinely four ultrasounds should be asked for in all pregnancies. The parameters to be checked in all four ultrasounds are mentioned. They are:

From 6-9 Weeks

- Uterine size
- Location of gestational sac
- Number of gestational sacs
- Size of gestational sac
- Yolk sac
- Size of yolk sac
- Embryo/fetus size
- Menstrual age
- Cardiac activity
- Heart rate
- Trophoblastic reaction
- Any uterine mass
- Any adnexal mass
- Corpus luteum (present/absent).

From 10-14 Weeks

- Placental site
- Liquor amnii
- Fetal crown rump length
- Menstrual age
- Fetal movements and cardiac activity
- Any gross anomalies
- Nuchal translucency
- Nasal bone (Present/absent)
- Ductus venosus flow
- Internal os width
- Length of cervix
- Any uterine mass
- Any adnexal mass.

From 18-22 Weeks

- Placenta
- Liquor amnii
- Umbilical cord
- Cervix
- Lower segment
- Myometrium
- Adnexa
- Nuchal skin thickness
- Cerebellar transverse diameter
- Cisterna magna depth
- Width of body of lateral ventricle
- Inter-hemispheric distance
- Ratio of the width of body of lateral ventricle to inter-hemispheric distance
- Ocular diameter
- Interocular distance
- Binocular distance

- Bi-parietal diameter
- Occipitofrontal distance
- Head perimeter
- Abdominal perimeter
- Femoral length
- Humeral length
- Foot length
- Fetal movements and cardiac activity
- Ductus venosus flow velocity waveform
- Both maternal uterine artery Doppler.

From 35-40 Weeks

- Placenta
- Liquor amnii
- Umbilical cord
- Cervix
- Lower segment
- Myometrium
- Adnexa
- Bi-parietal diameter
- Occipitofrontal distance
- Head perimeter
- Abdominal perimeter
- Femoral length
- Distal femoral epiphysis
- Biophysical profile/modified biophysical profile (AFI and VAST)
- Color Doppler arterial (Umbilical artery, middle cerebral artery, descending aorta and both maternal uterine arteries)
- Color Doppler venous (Umbilical vein, inferior vena cava and ductus venosus).

CHAPTER 2

Training

The practice of ultrasound and the use of diagnostic and interventional ultrasound is now a necessary tool rather than a luxury. It is impossible to even conceive an Obstetric Care Unit and Fetal Medicine Unit or even Gynecology and Infertility Diagnostic Unit without ultrasound.

To practise ultrasound in India it is mandatory to be trained in ultrasonography under proper guides and to do 100 cases minimum of Obs. Gyn. Ultrasound and 6 months of observership under a Radiologist or an approved center.

2.1 THEORETICAL ASPECTS

The theoretical aspects one should know, should cover topics on physics of ultrasound, ultrasound machines and probes, how to use an ultrasound machine, PNDT Act, laws of ultrasound, medicolegal aspects, methodology, patient preparations, complete obstetric ultrasound uses including use in first, second and third trimesters, diagnosis of threatened abortion, ectopic pregnancy, biometery, anomaly scanning, IUGR, placental evaluation, amniotic fluid evaluation, color Doppler uses and 3D and 4D ultrasound.

Complete gynecological ultrasound aspects include use of TVS, color and 3D in evaluating female pelvis and evaluating infertility and complete interventional procedures.

2.2 TRAINING PARAMETERS

First Level
(At Least 30 Hours a Week for Two Months)

These are aimed at:
1. Confirm intrauterine pregnancy.
2. Confirm viability.
3. Determine number of gestations.
4. Fetal biometry.
5. Assessment of growth.
6. Presentation.
7. Amniotic fluid assessment.
8. Placental assessment.
9. Cervix measurement.
10. Suspect abnormalities.

Second Level
(About 100 Sessions and 300 Hours)

These are aimed at:
1. Detect and specify early pregnancy problems.
2. Detect and specify abnormalities.
3. Assessment of growth restriction.
4. Fetal biophysical profiling.
5. Understanding color Doppler.
6. Accurately sampling various blood vessels by Doppler and analysing them.
7. Knowledge of interventional procedure.
8. Knowledge of 3 D and 4 D.
9. Analysis of malignancies.

Third Level (3 Years)

These are aimed at:
1. Acquiring 3 D and 4 D image.
2. Perform interventional procedures.
3. Research and development.
4. Ability to teach basic stalls.

2.3 SUGGESTED TRAINING SCHEDULE

Viable pregnancies	10
Nonviable pregnancies	10
Normal biometry	10
Growth restrictions	10
Abnormal pregnancy	10
(Ectopic/Multiple, etc.)	
Color Doppler studies obstetric	10
Gynec	10
IUCD's	5
Fibroids	10
Ovarian cysts	10
Gynec disorders	10
Transvaginal scan	10

These are minimum number of scans for Level I training.

Another 100 cases of detailed Obstetric and Gynecological cases for various indications including color and 3 D should be logged for Level II training.

A standard reporting format for gynecology and Obstetrics should be adhered to with details of different descriptive terminology.

2.4 PREREQUISITE CRITERIA FOR A TRAINED ULTRASONOLOGIST

1. The ultrasonologist should be able to identify early pregnancy and emergency gynecological problems by transvaginal and transabdominal ultrasound.

a. *Early pregnancy:*
  - Fetal viability
  - Description of the gestational sac, embryo, yolk sac
  - Single and multiple gestation (chorionicity).

b. *Pathology:*
  - Early pregnancy failure
  - Ectopic pregnancy
  - Gross fetal abnormalities such as nuchal translucency, hydropic abnormalities
  - Hydatidiform mole
  - Associated pelvic tumors.

c. *Gynecology:*
  - Normal pelvic anatomy
  - Uterine size and endometrial thickness
  - Measurement of ovaries
  - Pelvic tumors, e.g. fibroids, cysts hydrosalpinx
  - Peritoneal fluid
  - Intrauterine contraceptive devices.

2. The ultrasonologist should be able to recognise the following normal fetal anatomical features from 18 weeks onwards by abdominal ultrasound.

  a. *Shape of the skull:* Nuchal skinfold
  b. *Brain:* Ventricles and cerebellum, choroid plexus
  c. Facial profile
  d. *Spine:* Both longitudinally and transversely
  e. Heart rate and rhythm, size and position, four-chamber view
  f. Size and morphology of the lungs
  g. Shape of the thorax and abdomen
  h. *Abdomen:* Diaphragm, stomach, liver and umbilical vein, kidneys, abdominal wall and umbilicus
  i. *Limbs:* Femur, tibia and fibula, humerus, radius and ulna, feet and hands—these to include shape, echogenicity and movement

    j. *Multiple pregnancy:* Monochorionic and dischorionic, twin-twin transfusion syndrome

    k. Amount of amniotic fluid

    l. Placental location

    m. Cord and number of vessels.

3. *Fetal biometry*

    a. Crown rump length, biparietal diameter, femur length, head circumference, abdominal circumference, interpretation of growth charts.

4. *Activity:* Recognize and quantify

    a. Fetal movements

    b. Breathing movements

    c. Eye movements.

2.5 MANDATORY PROPOSED CERTIFICATION FOR AN ULTRASONOLOGIST (OBS. AND GYN.)

1. One hundred hours in 6 months, of supervised scanning to include (one year observership):

    a. 100 gynecological examinations and early pregnancy problems (principally by transvaginal sonography but transabdominal experience also required).

    b. 200 obstetric scans covering the full spectrum of obstetric conditions.

2. *Logbooks:* 30 cases on one A4 page with ultrasound picture, at least 15 anomalies should be included.

These are suggested training hours and comply with the Indian Government's requirement under the modified PNDT Act.

First Trimester

3.1 INDICATIONS

1. Confirmation of pregnancy
2. Vaginal bleeding in pregnancy (Threatened abortion)
3. Estimation of gestational age
4. Suspected ectopic pregnancy
5. Suspected hydatidiform mole
6. Adjunct to cervical cerclage

7. Suspected multiple gestation
8. Adjunct to chorionic villus sampling

3.2 NORMAL FIRST TRIMESTER EMBRYONIC/FETAL EVALUATION

1. Location of sac:
   a. Fundus (Fig. 3.1)
   b. Corpus (Fig. 3.2)
   c. Cornual (Fig. 3.3)
   d. Superior to the cervix
2. Number of sacs:
   a. Single
   b. Multiple (Twin/triplet/high order multiple) (Fig. 3.4)
3. Size of sac:
   a. In toto, measure inner to inner diameter of gestational sac on all three sides and calculate the size and corresponding gestational age (Fig. 3.5).
   b. Size of gestational sac in comparison to the embryo/fetus size (Fig. 3.6).
4. Embryo/fetal size (Crown rump length) (Figs 3.7 and 3.8)
5. Embryonic cardiac activity. To begin with, the heart rate is around 85 beats/minute at 5 to 5½ weeks (Fig. 3.9) increasing to around 160 beats/minute (Fig. 3.10) at nine weeks.
6. Yolk sac
   a. Size
   b. Shape
   c. Any calcification
7. Trophoblastic reaction:
   a. Whether wrapping around and thick reaction (Fig. 3.11)
   b. Locate site (Fig. 3.12)

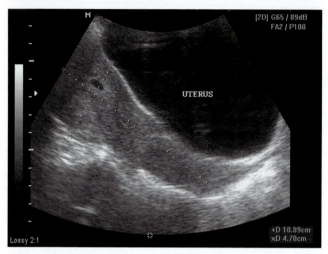

Fig. 3.1: Gestational sac located in the uterine fundus

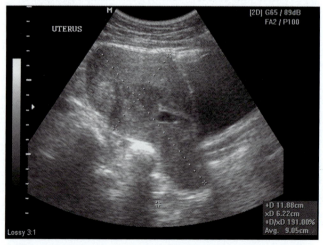

Fig. 3.2: Gestational sac located in the uterine corpus

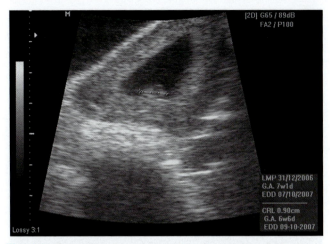

Fig. 3.3: Gestational sac located in the uterine cavity in the cornual area. Note the amount of myometrium lateral to the gestational sac differentiating it from a cornual ectopic

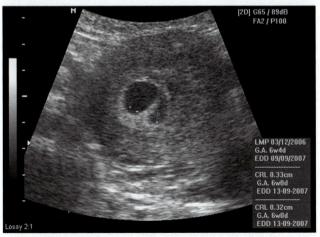

Fig. 3.4: Two gestational sacs both located in the uterine fundus

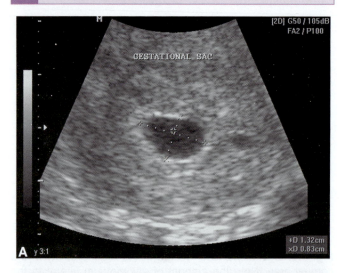

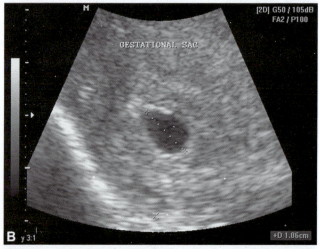

Figs 3.5A and B: Gestational sac measurement in all three planes and calculation of gestational age done by the ultrasound machine

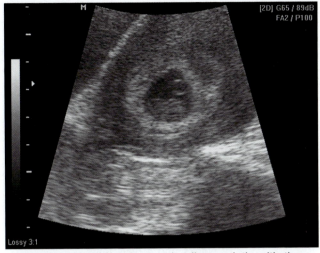

Fig. 3.6: Note that the sac is oligoamniotic with the gestational sac corresponding less than the embryo size

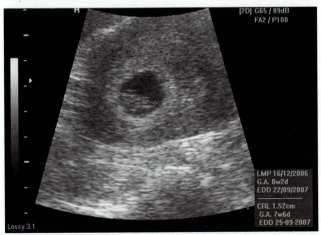

Fig. 3.7: Measurement of crown rump length in a 7 weeks and 6 days embryo

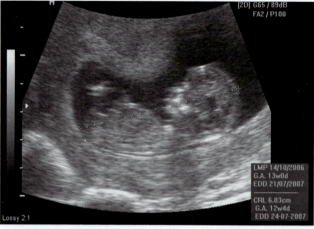

Fig. 3.8: Measurement of crown rump length in an 12 weeks and 4 days fetus

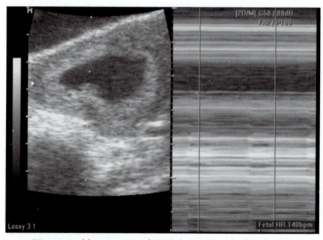

Fig. 3.9: Heart rate of 143 beats per minute in a 6 weeks and 0 days embryo

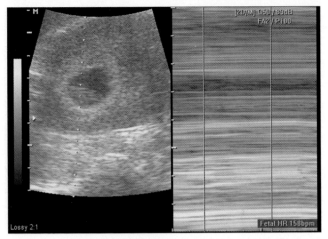

Fig. 3.10: Heart rate of 151 beats per minute in an 8 weeks and 1 day fetus

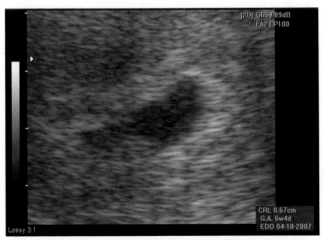

Fig. 3.11: Wrapping around thick trophoblastic reaction seen in a gestational sac of 6 weeks 4 days

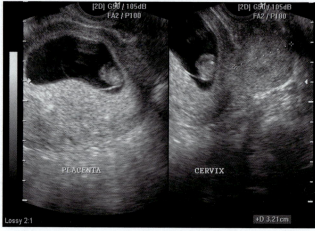

Fig. 3.12: Note the thickened trophoblastic echoes on one wall of the gestational sac. This is the placental site location

8. Separation:
   a. Amnio-decidual separation (Fig. 3.13)
   b. Chorio-decidual separation (Fig. 3.14)
9. To identify any gross anomalies
   a. Gross abnormalities of the cranium, spine, abdomen and limbs can be detected even in the late first trimester.
   b. Nasal bone ossification
   c. Nuchal translucency
10. Color Doppler evaluation of the ductus venosus and both maternal uterine arteries

3.3 NORMAL PARAMETER EVALUATION IN THE FIRST TRIMESTER

1. *Gestational sac:* Seen as early as 4½ weeks by transvaginal scan and 5½weeks by transabdominal scan (Fig. 3.15).

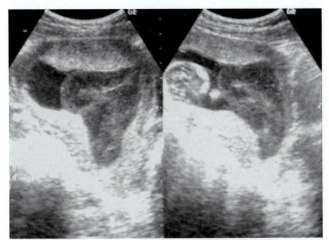

Fig. 3.13: The placenta is anterior with an amnio-decidual separation seen in the anterior wall superior to the cervix. This has an associated collection of 8.35 ml

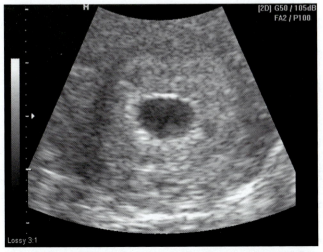

Fig. 3.14: Multiple foci of chorio-decidual separation seen in a 6-7 weeks size missed abortion

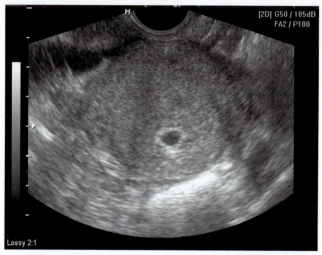

Fig. 3.15: Transvaginal scan of a gestational sac of 5 weeks size

2. *Yolk sac:* Seen as early as 5 weeks by transvaginal scan and 6 weeks by transabdominal scan (Fig. 3.16).
3. *Embryo:* Seen at 5½ weeks by transvaginal scan and at 6-6½ weeks by transabdominal scan (Fig. 3.17).
4. *Cardiac activity:* Appears at 5 weeks and 4 days.

3.4 ABNORMAL INTRAUTERINE PREGNANCY

1. No embryonic cardiac activity with a CRL > 5 mm. (Missed abortion) (Fig. 3.18).
2. Gestational sac larger than 8 mm without a yolk sac. (Blighted ovum) (Fig. 3.19).
3. Gestational sac larger than 16 mm without an embryo. (Anembryonic pregnancy) (Fig. 3.20).
4. Abnormally large or irregular or small amniotic sac (Fig. 3.21).

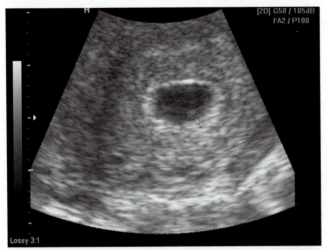

Fig. 3.16: Gestational sac of 5 weeks and 2 days with a yolk sac clearly delineated

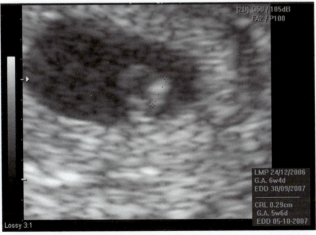

Fig. 3.17: Pregnancy of 5 weeks and 6 days gestation showing a yolk sac and an embryo

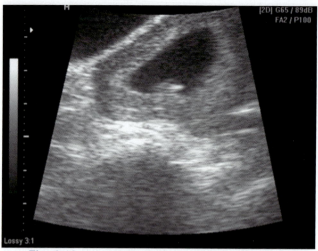

Fig. 3.18: No cardiac activity seen in this 8 mm pulseless attenuated embryo

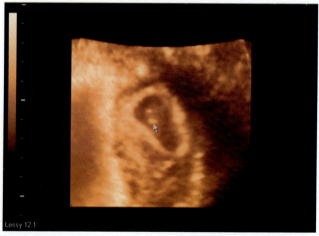

Fig. 3.19: Thin-walled irregular gestational sac of 15 mm in the uterine fundus with a pulseless embryo

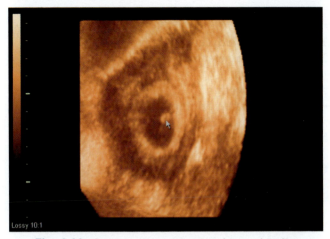

Fig. 3.20: Seven weeks gestational sac showing a yolk sac but no embryo

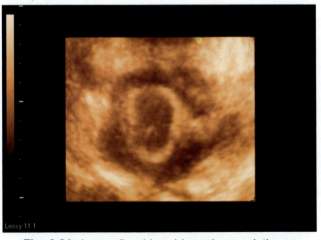

Fig. 3.21: Large, flaccid and irregular amniotic sac with a pulseless embryo

3.5 IMPENDING EARLY PREGNANCY FAILURE

1. Embryonic bradycardia relative to CRL.
2. Mean sac diameter minus CRL is less than 5 mm (oligo-amniotic sac).
3. Poor sac growth.
4. Large (> 5.6 mm prior to 10 weeks)/abnormal yolk sac (Figs 3.22 and 3.23).
5. Disappearance of the corpus luteum.

Classification of Early Pregnancy Loss

Stage A:
- Loss withing first 2 weeks
- Subclinical loss
- No sonographic evidence

Stage B:
- Loss at 5-6 weeks
- Empty gestational sac

Stage C:
- Loss at 7-8 weeks
- Abnormal gestational sac and embryo

Stage D:
- Loss at 9-12 weeks
- Abnormal embryo.

3.6 ECTOPIC GESTATION

1. Demonstration of live embryo in the adnexa is diagnostic of ectopic pregnancy (Fig. 3.24).
2. Nonspecific findings of an ectopic pregnancy are an adnexal mass (Fig. 3.23), free fluid (Fig. 3.25), a tubal ring (Fig. 3.26) and identification of adnexal peritrophoblastic flow (Fig. 3.27).
3. Vascular ring can be delineated (Fig. 3.28).

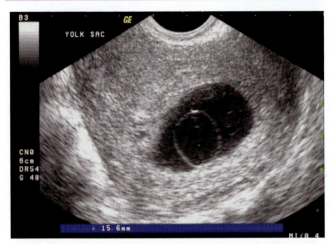

Fig. 3.22: Large yolk sac with the
embryo seen adjacent to it

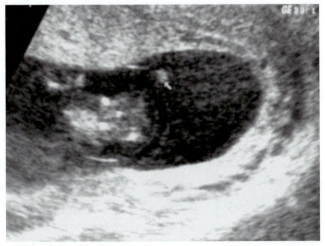

Fig. 3.23: Shrunken yolk sac with an extensive cystic
hygroma associated with it

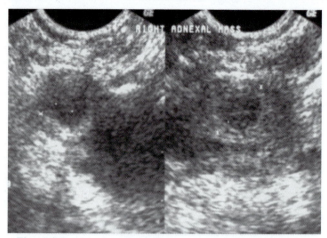

Fig. 3.24: Live ectopic with a gestational sac, yolk sac and an embryo with cardiac activity

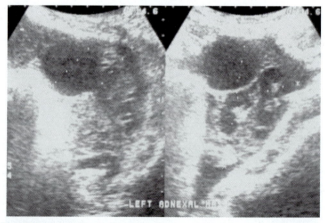

Fig. 3.25: Left adnexal mass with corpus luteum in the left ovary with an adjacent inhomogeneous adnexal mass and peri-lesional fluid collection

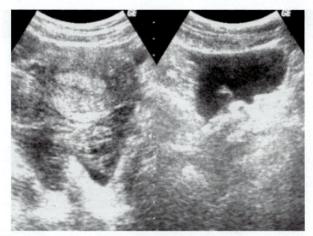

Fig. 3.26: Adnexal mass with free fluid (pelvic hematocele) in the pouch of Douglas

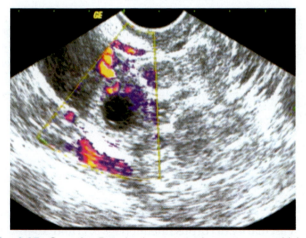

Fig. 3.27: On color Doppler in an ectopic pregnancy which is unruptured with viable trophoblasts a vascular ring is delineated with the blood flow characteristically showing low-impedance, high-diastolic flow

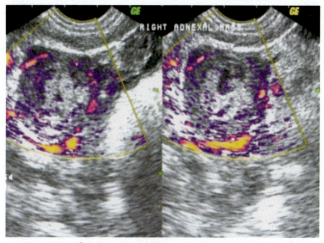

Fig. 3.28: Same case with marked peri-trophoblastic vascularity in the mass

4. The blood flow characteristically shows low-impedance, high-diastolic flow.
5. Intrauterine peri-trophoblastic flow is not seen and peri-endometrial venous flow is also very less.
6. Corpus luteal flow is identified in one or both ovaries.

3.7 EXTRA-FETAL EVALUATION

1. Myometrium (Fig. 3.29)
2. Cervical length (Fig. 3.30)
3. Internal os
4. Adnexal mass (Fig. 3.31)
5. Site of corpus luteum (Fig. 3.32)
6. Vascularity of corpus luteum (Figs 3.33 and 3.34).

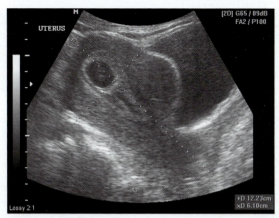

Fig. 3.29: Look for any masses in the myometrium. Early pregnancy with a posterior wall subserous fibroid. If you locate any fibroid specify the site (uterine or cervical) and the type (submucous, interstitial, subserous or panmural) so as to assess later in serial scans

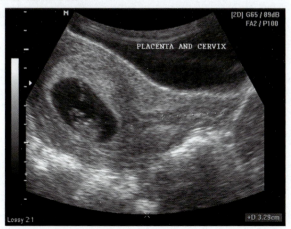

Fig. 3.30: Even in the first trimester always evaluate the cervical length by measuring from the cervical waist or the location of the internal os till the portion where the mucus plug ends. Any herniation or shortening to be reported for serial evaluation

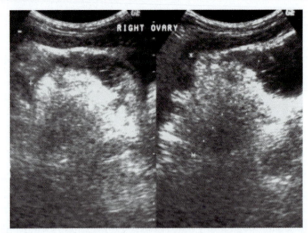

Fig. 3.31: Apart from the corpus luteum always evaluate the adnexa for any masses like dermoid, broad ligament fibroid or any other ovarian masses

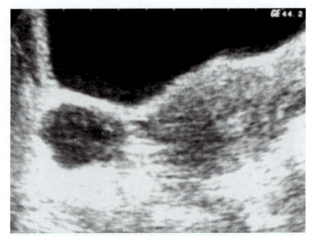

Fig. 3.32: Locate the corpus luteum as to which ovary it is in. Corpus luteum can appear iso- or hypoechoic within the ovary depending on hemorrhage

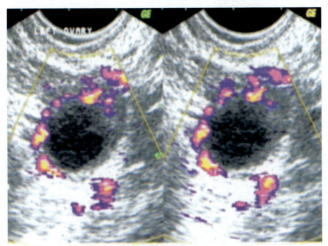

Fig. 3.33: On color flow mapping one can assess the vascularity of the corpus luteum

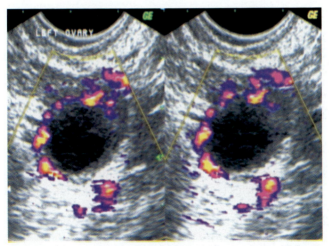

Fig. 3.34: Evaluate the vascularity of the corpus luteum by color flow mapping and the arterial flow velocity waveform on duplex Doppler should normally show a resistive index of less than 0.55

3.8 ABNORMAL INTRAUTERINE PREGNANCY FORMS

1. Threatened/missed abortion
2. Incomplete abortion
3. Complete abortion
4. Hydatiform mole
5. Blighted ovum.

3.9 COMPLETE ABORTION

1. No intrauterine gestational sac seen (empty uterus sign)
2. Cavity echoes are thin and usually homogeneous (Fig. 3.35)
3. Uterine vascularity is cold or warm (Fig. 3.36)
4. There is minimal or absent intrauterine peri-trophoblastic flow (Fig. 3.37)
5. Intrauterine venous flow is minimal or absent.

3.10 INCOMPLETE ABORTION

1. Inhomogeneous cavity echoes (Fig. 3.38)
2. Overall uterine vascularity diffusely increased (warm or hot vascularity) (Fig. 3.39)
3. Peri-trophoblastic arterial flow present with high systolic velocities (Fig. 3.40)
4. Peri-endometrial venous flow also increased (Fig. 3.41).

3.11 MOLAR CHANGE

1. Echogenic tissue interspersed with numerous punctate sonolucencies (snow storm appearance) (Figs 3.42 and 3.43)
2. In uncomplicated cases only mild increase in peri-lesional vascularity is noted
3. In invasive moles very high velocity flow in areas of tumor invasion within the myometrium are seen (Fig. 3.44).

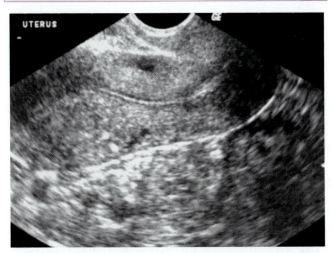

Fig. 3.35: A case of complete spontaneous abortion with very thin cavity echoes, 3-4 mm

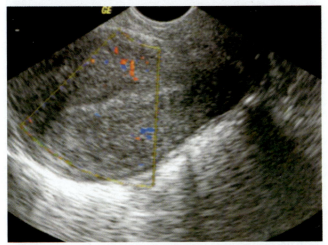

Fig. 3.36: The uterine vascularity is usually cold in a case of complete spontaneous abortion

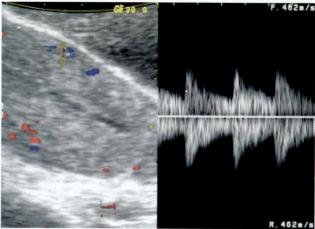

Fig. 3.37: Intrauterine peri-trophoblastic flow is not seen and only peripheral myometrial vascularity seen

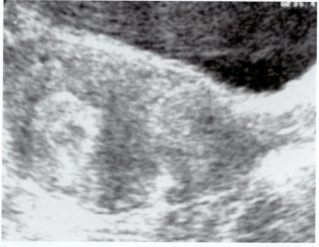

Fig. 3.38: Inhomogeneous echoes within the uterine cavity seen on 2D ultrasound in a case of amenorrhea 6 weeks with bleeding for 3 days

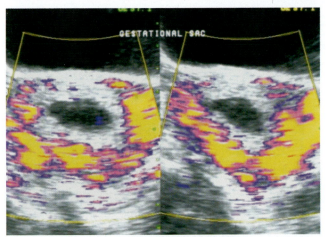

Fig. 3.39: Case of missed abortion seen on 2D ultrasound and on color Doppler, the overall uterine vascularity is increased (warm or hot vascularity)

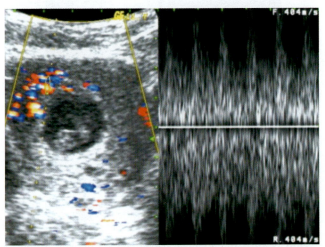

Fig. 3.40: Same case on duplex Doppler evaluation the peritrophoblastic arterial flow is identified, with systolic velocities much above the normal range for intrauterine pregnancy

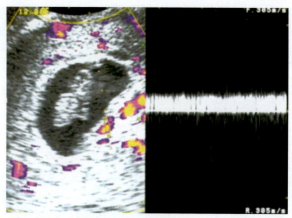

Fig. 3.41: Case of missed abortion with increased peri-endometrial venous flow

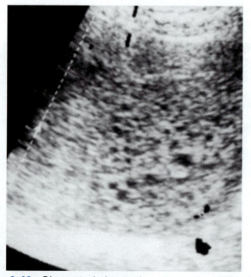

Fig. 3.42: Characteristic cystic spaces packed in the uterine cavity are seen in this case of molar pregnancy

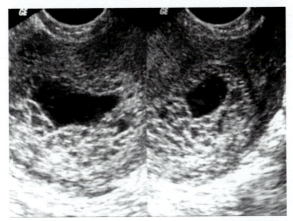

Fig. 3.43: Nonviable gestational sac with thin-walled clear cystic spaces around the gestational sac

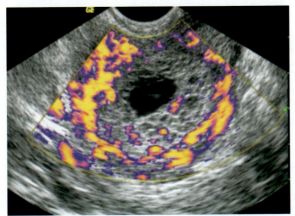

Fig. 3.44: In molar pregnancy in uncomplicated cases only mild increase in peri-lesional vascularity is noted. In invasive moles very high velocity flow in areas of tumor invasion within the myometrium are seen. Very low impedance flow with almost an arteriovenous shunt type waveform is also seen. This hypervascularity recedes with regression of the tumor

3.12 SONO-EMBRYOLOGY CHART
(FIGS 3.45 TO 3.55)

Date	Event	Sonological evaluation
Day 14	Ovulation	Collapse of follicle, free fluid, corpus luteum, Secretory endometrium
Day 15	Fertilization	—
Day 18	Morula stage	Decidualization of endometrium
Day 22-23	Blastocyst	Implantation window
Day 23	Primary yolk sac	Implantation site
Day 26-28	Extra embryonic Coelom	Implantation site recognition
Day 27-28	Secondary yolk sac	
Day 28	Syncytiotrophoblast and sometimes seen Chorionic cavity	
Week 5 29/30	Gastrulation	Visualization of gestational sac, and secondary, yolk sac
31/42	Neuralization	Growth of sac embryo Fetal cardiac activity
34/44	Somites	Embryo visualization Crown rump length Cardiac activity
Week 6-12	Cardiovascular system	—
6 weeks	Unidirectional blood flow	Cardiac activity
8 weeks	Heart/	Seen by TVS
10 weeks	Peripheral vascular system	Visualized

Contd...

Contd...

Gastrointestinal tract

6 weeks	Primitive Gut	
8-12 weeks	Gut lies outside in umbilical cord	Physiological herniation

Genitourinary

8 weeks	Primitive kidney	Not yet seen
11 weeks	Kidney develops urine production	Seen Bladder seen
14 weeks	External genitalia	Can be seen

Musculoskeletal system

6 weeks	Limb buds	Can be seen
8 weeks	Digital rays	Can be seen
	Clavide ossification	Seen
9 weeks	Mandible ossification	Seen
10 weeks	Nasal bone ossification	Seen
10 weeks	Spinal ossification	Spine seen
11 weeks	Frontal bones	
11 weeks	Long bone ossification	

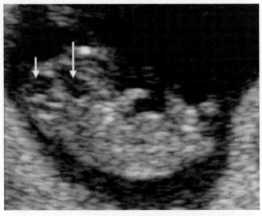

Fig. 3.45: Anechoic areas (arrows) seen in the brain of a fetus of 9 weeks and 6 days

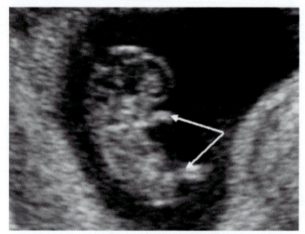

Fig. 3.46: Upper and lower limbs (arrows) seen

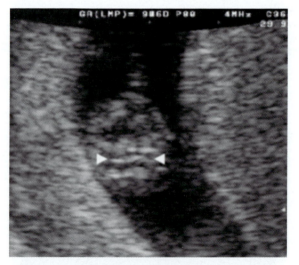

Fig. 3.47: Cerebellar hemispheres (arrow heads)
with deficiency in the vermis (physiological at this stage)

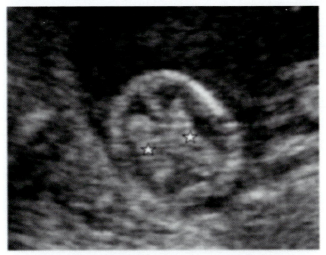

Fig. 3.48: Echogenic choroid plexii (stars) in the lateral ventricles

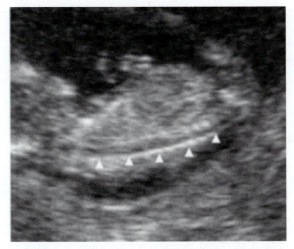

Fig. 3.49: Fetal spine can be seen as two parallel lines

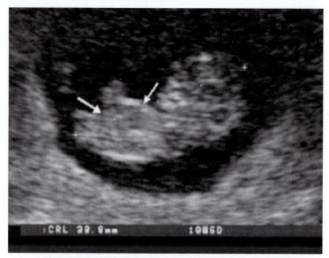

Fig. 3.50: Physiological herniation (arrows) of bowel seen below the umbilical cord

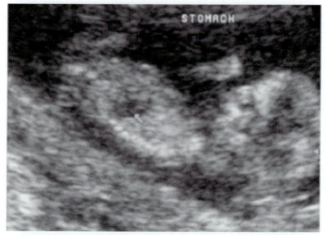

Fig. 3.51: Fetal stomach bubble seen in a fetus of 11 weeks and 4 days

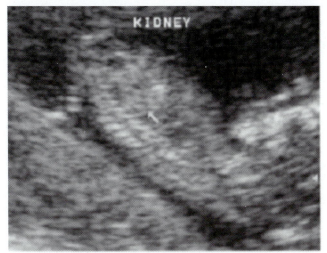

Fig. 3.52: Fetal kidney seen as an echogenic structure adjacent to the fetal spine

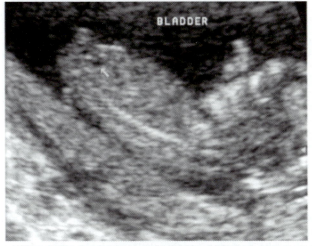

Fig. 3.53: Fetal urinary bladder seen in a fetus of 12 weeks and 2 days

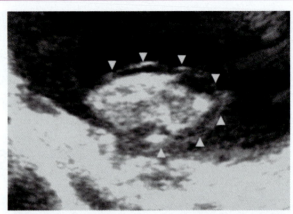

Fig. 3.54: Extensive cystic hygroma (arrow heads) in a 10 weeks and 1 day fetus

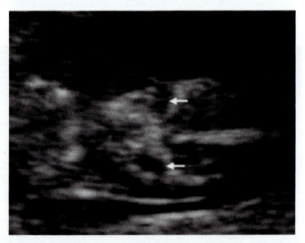

Fig. 3.55: Orbits (arrows) delineated as early as 11 weeks. Measure the ocular diameter, interocular distance and binocular distance to diagnose hypotelorism. Visualization of both orbits excludes anophthalmia or single orbit deformity

Table 3.1: Ultrasound appearances of an early pregnancy failure

1. > 5 mm embryo without cardiac activity (Fig. 3.56)
2. > 8 mm gestational sac without a yolk sac (Fig. 3.57)
3. >16 mm gestational sac without an embryo (Fig. 3.58)
4. Flaccid, large or irregular amniotic sac (Fig. 3.59)

Table 3.2: Ultrasound appearances of an impending early pregnancy failure

1. Embryonic bradycardia in relation with the gestational age
2. Oligo-amniotic sac (Fig. 3.60)
3. Interval sac growth poor
4. Abnormal shape or size of yolk sac (Figs 3.61 and 3.62)

Table 3.3: Embryonic time table and its appearances on ultrasound

Structures visible on ultrasound	No. of weeks from last menstrual period
Gestational sac	4w4d-5w0d
Yolk sac	5w0d-5w3d
Embryonic pole	5w2d
Cardiac pulsations	5w3d
Limb buds	8w0d and >
Fetal movements	8w0d and >
Bowel herniation	9w0d-11w0d
Kidneys	10w0d and >
Choroid plexus	10w0d and >
Calcification of calvarium	10w0d and >
Orbits	10w4d and >
Stomach bubble	11w0d and >
Cardiac configuration	12w0d and >
Urinary bladder	12w0d and >

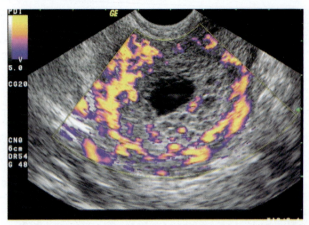

Fig. 3.56: Embryo 7 mm in size with no cardiac activity. Note the increase in peri-trophoblastic vascularity which further helps in the diagnosis of an unhealthy pregnancy

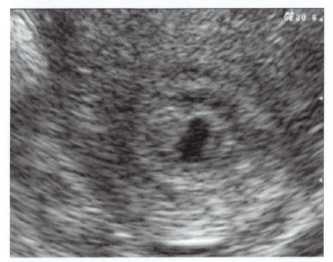

Fig. 3.57: Gestational sac, 12 mm in size without a yolk sac or a fetal node

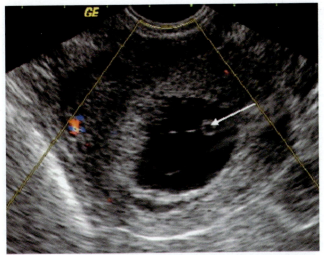

Fig. 3.58: Gestational sac, 26 mm in size with a yolk sac (arrow) but with no fetal node seen

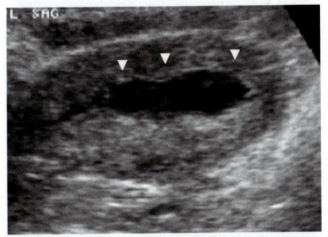

Fig. 3.59: Thin-walled, irregular and flaccid gestational sac of 7-8 weeks size with no yolk sac or embryo seen. Note the multiple foci of chorio-decidual separation (arrow heads)

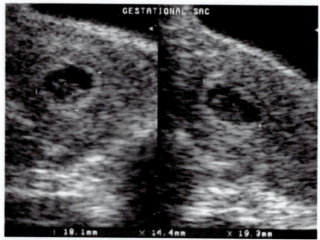

Fig. 3.60: Pregnancy of 7 weeks and 5 days showing an oligo-amniotic sac. The gestational sac size is 6 weeks and 2 days and the embryo size is 7 weeks and 4 days. The mean sac diameter is 17 mm and the crown rump length is 9 mm

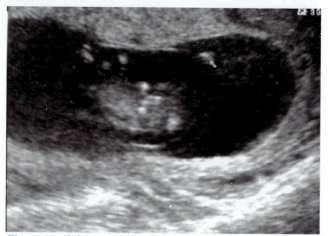

Fig. 3.61: A hyperechoic shrunken yolk sac on one side with a cystic hygroma of the fetus seen as well

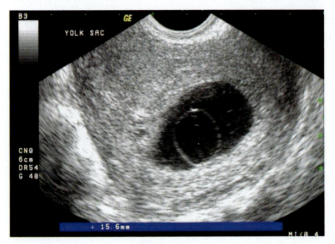

Fig. 3.62: Large yolk sec (15.6 mm) seen in the gestational sec

4. Very low impedance flow with almost an arteriovenous shunt type waveform is also seen.
5. Hypervascularity recedes with regression of the tumor.

3.13 NUCHAL TRANSLUCENCY

- In 74-77 percent of trisomy 21 fetuses the fetal nuchal translucency is increased with a low false- positive rate.
- Sensitivity for detection of chromosomal abnormalities is extremely high by a combined screening of maternal age, fetal-nuchal translucency, nasal bone, ductus venosus and maternal biochemistry.
- The translucency (subcutaneous) between the skin and soft tissue posterior to the cervical spine has to be measured (Fig. 3.63).
- Nuchal translucency thickness usually increases with gestational age with 1.5 mm and 2.5 mm being the 50th

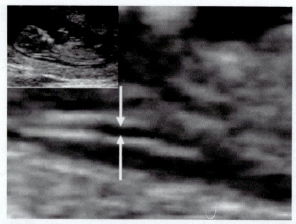

Fig. 3.63: The translucency (arrows) (subcutaneous) between the skin and soft tissue posterior to the cervical spine has to be measured

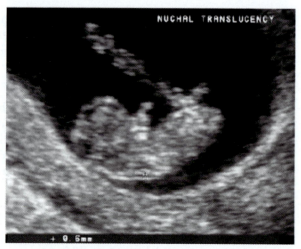

Fig. 3.64: Nuchal translucency thickness measurement in a 10 weeks size fetus

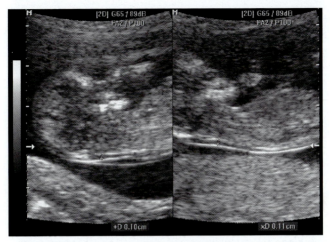

Fig. 3.65: Nuchal translucency thickness measurement in a 12 weeks size fetus

and 95th percentile respectively for gestational ages between 10 and 12 weeks. 2.0 mm and 21.0 mm are the 50th and 95th percentile respectively for gestational ages between 12 and 14 weeks (Figs 3.64 and 3.65).

- An increased nuchal translucency thickness (Figs 3.66 to 3.70) not only indicates increased suspicion of chromosomal abnormalities but also indicates a possibility of multiple structural defects especially of the fetal heart and abdomen. Therefore, a normal karyotype does not in any way ensure normalcy of the fetus.
- A thickened nuchal translucency with spontaneous resolution and a normal nuchal skin fold thickness does not exclude a karyotypic abnormality.
- High risk patients for chromosomal abnormalities and cardiac defects should definitely be subjected to an ultrasound between 10 and 14 weeks for measurement of nuchal translucency thickness.

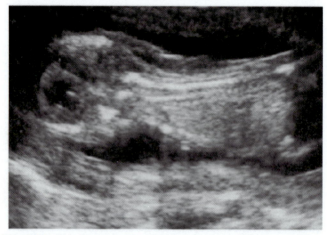

Fig. 3.66: The fetus showed an increased nuchal translucency thickness (0.5 mm at 12 weeks). An early amniocentesis showed a Trisomy 21 karyotype

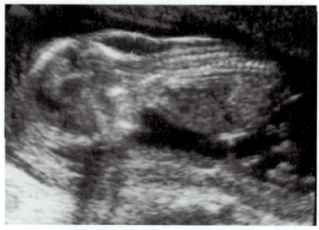

Fig. 3.67: Increased nuchal translucency thickness (6 mm at 13 weeks and 1 day)

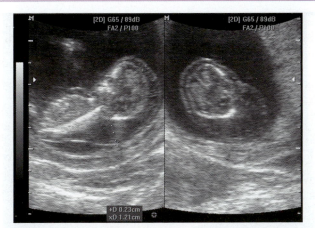

Fig. 3.68: Increased nuchal translucency thickness (5 mm at 12 weeks and 5 days). Patient refused an amniocentesis. Detailed anomaly scanning and fetal echocardiography at 18 weeks showed a transposition of great vessels

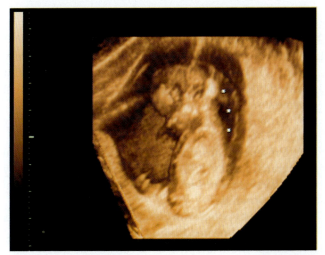

Fig. 3.69: Increased nuchal translucency as seen on 3D

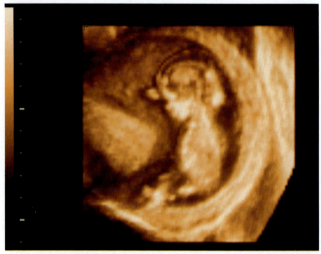

Fig. 3.70: Thickened nuchal translucency as seen on 3D

3.14 ABNORMAL FETUS

1. Fetal abnormalities like Acrania (Fig. 3.71), Anencephaly (Fig. 3.72), Limb reduction defects, Gross anterior abdominal wall defects can be diagnosed in the late first trimester.
   - Proboscis can be delineated on ultrasound as early as 12 weeks.
   - Presence or absence of nasal bone along with nuchal translucency and ductus venosus flow velocity waveform are sensitive markers for chromosomal abnormalities.
   - Severe hypotelorism can also be delineated as orbits can be delineated from 11 weeks onwards.
   - Single orbit, anophthalmia can also be diagnosed.

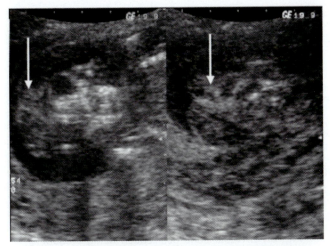

Fig. 3.71: Case of acrania with only brain and no bone seen superior to the orbits

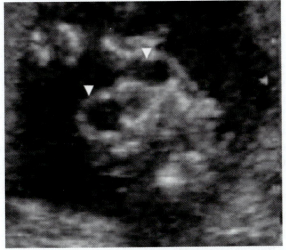

Fig. 3.72: Case of anencephaly with no brain or bone seen superior to the orbits

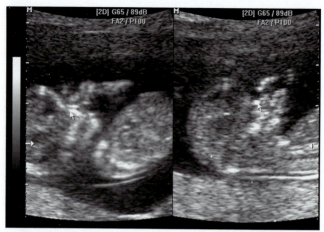

Fig. 3.73: Nasal bone ossification being present or absent is a marker for Trisomies especially Trisomy 21

2. Nasal bone ossification (Fig. 3.73) being absent can be diagnosed in the first trimester to raise the suspicion of chromosomal abnormalities.
3. Thickened nuchal translucency can again raise the suspicion of chromosomal abnormalities and one can go in for early amniocentesis or biochemical markers to diagnose them. If nuchal translucency thickness resolves it does not indicate normalcy and on an amniocentesis if karyotype is normal subject the fetus to an echocardiography as an increased nuchal translucency thickness can denote a cardiac abnormality as well.

3.15 FIRST TRIMESTER SCAN CHECKLIST

1. LMP and gestation.
2. Identify uterus and gestational sac do not hesitate to do a transvaginal scan.

3. Confirm viability and number.
4. Look at the cervix and implantation site.
5. Check adnexa.
6. Measure embryo.
7. Give a sonological gestational age and EDD and verify with LMP.
8. Give a complete structured report with hard copy of pictures.

3.16 DILEMMAS

1. *Overdue:* Ultrasound or urine test. Urine test is positive before a gestational sac can be seen on an ultrasound scan.
2. *Urine test negative:* Ultrasound y/n. Definitely to rule out any ectopic gestation and to confirm the cause for the delayed period.
3. *Miscarried last time:* Should ultrasound be done. To be done to insure fetal well being and to discern any cause on ultrasound for recurrent pregnancy loss.
4. *Pain abdomen:* Ectopic will be definitely ruled out by ultrasound normally some or the other sign of ectopic pregnancy can be seen on an ultrasound scan, but many a times with overlapping nonspecific signs it can also be missed.

3.17 FIRST TRIMESTER KEY POINTS

- CRL = 10 mm = mean for 7 weeks
- CRL = 30 mm = mean for 9 weeks 5 days
- CRL = 60 mm = mean for 12 weeks 3 days
- A viable intrauterine pregnancy practically rules out ectopic gestation (Except one in 30000)
- There is a delay of identifying of one week by transabdominal as compared to transvaginal

Sac (2-4 mm)	4.5 weeks	5.5 weeks
Fetal heart (CRL2-4)	5 weeks	6 weeks
Yolk sac (10 mm)	5 weeks	6 weeks

- Early fetal bradycardia signifies poor prognosis
- Fetal chromosomal anomalies can be screened for and detected in the 10-14 weeks scan
- Transvaginal scan does not increase abortion risk of bleeding
- A thorough knowledge of fetal embryology and implantation and corpus luteum physiology is a must for first trimester diagnosis
- Do not hesitate to take second opinion
- 20 mm sac with no intra sac structures is suggestive of anembryonic pregnancy. A CRL of > 6 mm without fetal heart is suggestive of missed abortion. Confirm by TVS and repeat scan if required.

3.18 TRANSVAGINAL DECISION FLOW CHART

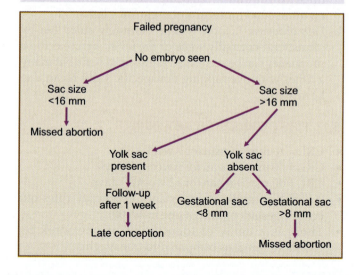

3.19 DECISION MAKING IN THE FIRST TRIMESTER

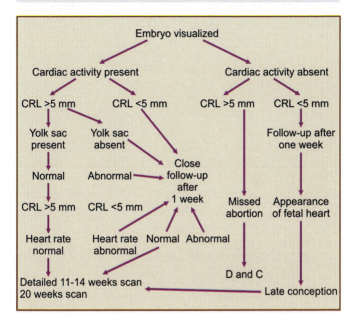

Second Trimester

4.1 INDICATIONS

1. Follow-up observation of identified fetal anomaly or history of previous congenital anomaly
2. Adjunct to amniocentesis
3. Abnormal serum alpha-fetoprotein value
4. Suspected polyhydramnios or oligohydramnios
5. Advanced maternal age
6. Exposure to drugs/radiation
7. Maternal diabetes mellitus
8. Bad obstetric history.

Scanning is done with a fully distended maternal bladder, though this is not essential after 20 weeks.

4.2 FETAL EVALUATION

1. Number
2. Fetal position especially in the late second trimester
3. Viability
4. Movements
5. Gestational age
6. Biometry.

4.3 FETAL EVALUATION (MALFORMATIONS)

The ideal way is to do a basic survey of fetal anatomy done systematically followed by a targeted fetal anatomy survey.
1. Cranium
2. Spine
3. Neck
4. Face
5. Thorax and heart
6. Abdomen
7. Extremities

4.4 CRANIUM (FIGS 4.1 TO 4.26)

1. Skull
2. Brain
3. Choroid plexus
   a. Cysts
   b. Hydrocephalus
4. Posterior cranial fossa
   a. Cerebellar transverse diameter
   b. Depth of cisterna magna
   c. Superior and inferior cerebellar vermis
   d. Posterior fossa cyst
   e. Communication between fourth ventricle and cisterna magna.

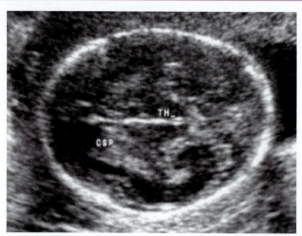

Fig. 4.1: Section for cranial biometry consisting of the thalamus, the third ventricle and the cavum septum pellucidum. The biparietal diameter is the side to side measurement from the outer table of the proximal skull to the inner table of the distal skull. The head perimeter is the the total cranial circumference, which includes the maximum anteroposterior diameter. The occipito-frontal diameter is the front to back measurement from the outer table on both sides

4.5 NUCHAL SKIN (FIGS 4.27 TO 4.32)

1. Thickness
2. Septations.

4.6 FETAL ORBITS AND FACE (FIGS 4.33 TO 4.47)

1. Hypo and hypertelorism
2. Lips
3. Lens
4. Nostrils
5. Ear.

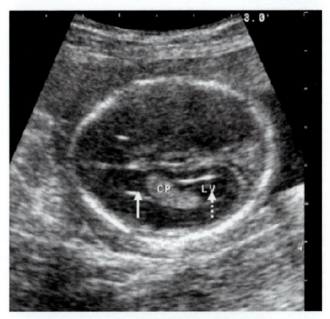

Fig. 4.2: Choroid plexus (CP) seen occupying the whole of the body of the lateral ventricle (LV). The anterior horn of the lateral ventricle (solid arrow) seen on the left side and posterior horn of the lateral ventricle (dashed arrow) seen on the right side are not filled by the choroid plexus.The choroid plexus quite often does not occupy the whole of the body of the lateral ventricle and the frontal and the posterior horn also are not filled by the choroids plexus. The width of the body of the lateral ventricle, the inter-hemispheric distance and the ratio of the width of the body of the lateral ventricle to the inter-hemispheric distance is calculated. (Normal value < 50%). This is not sensitive for early hydrocephalus. The width of the body, anterior horn and posterior horn of the lateral ventricle are taken (Normal value < 8 mm, Borderline 8-10 mm and > 10 mm abnormal)

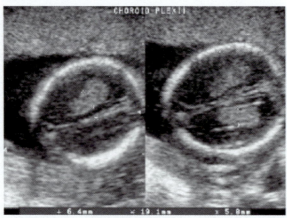

Fig. 4.3: When the choroid plexus does not occupy the whole of the body of the lateral ventricle see for the measurement of the medial separation of the choroid plexus from the wall of the lateral ventricle (Normal value < 2 mm, Borderline 2-3 mm and > 3 mm is abnormal)

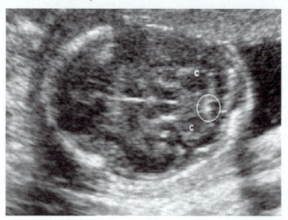

Fig. 4.4: The cerebellum is seen as a 'W' turned 90 degrees. The cerebellar hemispheres (C) and the cerebellar vermis (within the circle) should be appreciated for posterior cranial fossa abnormalities

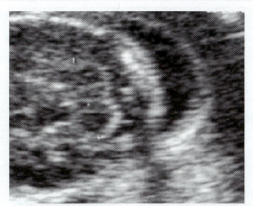

Fig. 4.5: The cerebellar transverse diameter (CTD) is measured from the edges of both cerebellar hemispheres. The CTD in mm from 14-22 weeks is equal to the gestational age of the fetus in weeks

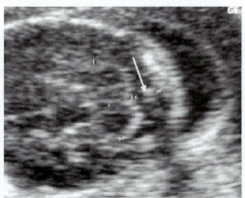

Fig. 4.6: The cisterna magna is seen posterior to the cerebellar vermis and anterior to the occipital bone (arrow). (Normal value < 8 mm, Borderline 8-10 mm and > 10 mm abnormal). Few strands seen traversing the cisterna magna are normal. Carefully check for any communication between the fourth ventricle and the cisterna magna with an abnormal cerebellar vermis. If there is any communication at gestational age less than 16 weeks revaluate the fetus after 2 weeks

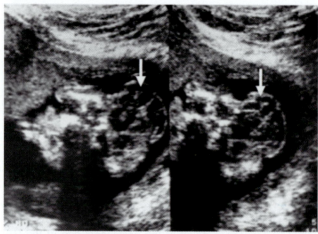

Fig. 4.7: Deformed cranium with almost no osseous area surrounding the floating brain (arrow)

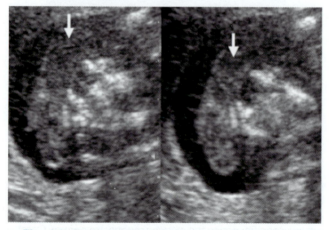

Fig. 4.8: Fetal acrania. Note the brain tissue (arrow) but no osseous covering over it

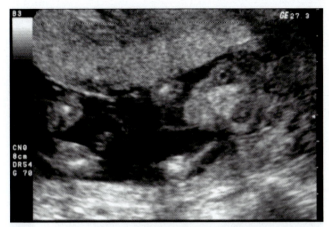

Fig. 4.9: Orbits seen with nothing
seen superior to it (neither brain nor bone)

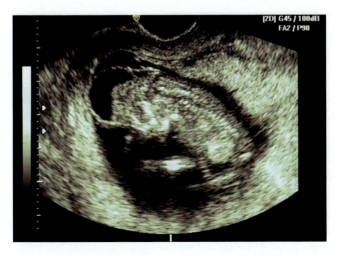

Fig. 4.10: Anencephaly: Superior to the orbits no
brain tissue or osseous portion is seen

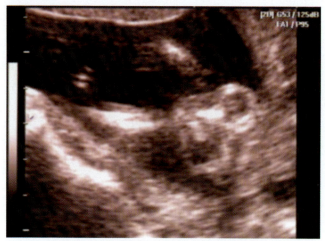

Fig. 4.11: Anencephaly with Toad sign

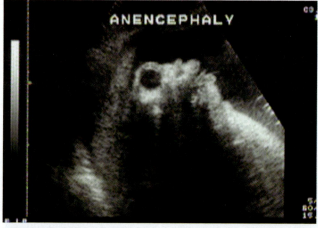

Fig. 4.12: Anencephaly with nothing superior to the orbits

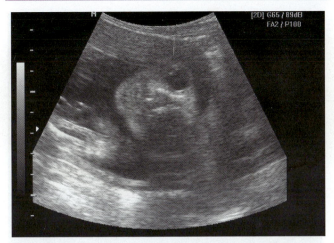

Fig. 4.13: Fetal face in an anencephalic fetus

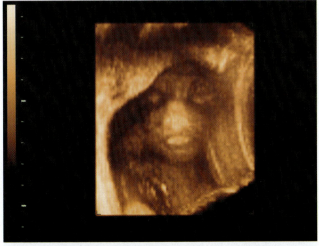

Fig. 4.14: Anencephaly as seen on 3D

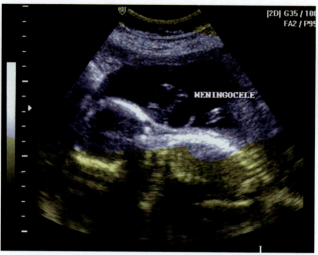

Fig. 4.15: Lateral occipital meningocele. Note the clear contents within the herniated sac

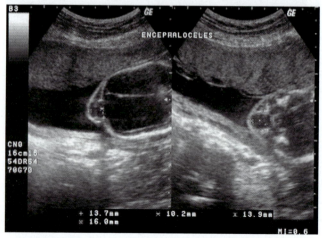

Fig. 4.16: Note the defect in the occipital bone with the herniation of brain tissue from the defect

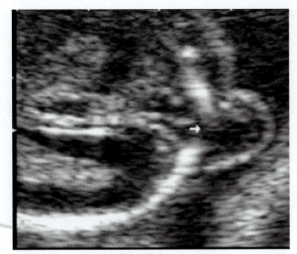

Fig. 4.17: Note the defect in the occipital bone (arrow) with the herniation of brain tissue from the defect

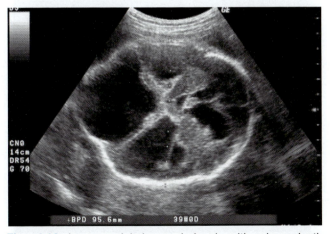

Fig. 4.18: Large occipital encephalocele with a hypoplastic cerebellar vermis

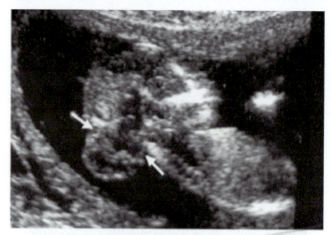

Fig. 4.19: Herniated contents (arrows) overhanging the fetal neck

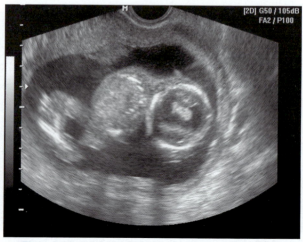

Fig. 4.20: Iniencephaly with a fixed retroflexion deformity of the fetal head

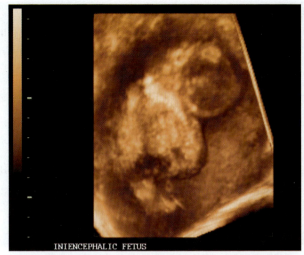

Fig. 4.21: Iniencephaly as seen on 3D

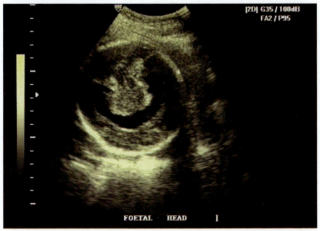

Fig. 4.22: Alobar holoprosencephaly with a dorsal sac and a monoventricular cavity with a displaced cerebral cortex

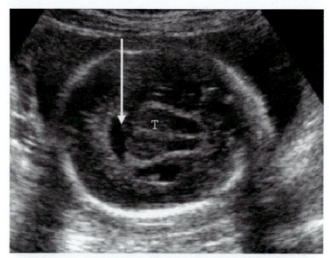

Fig. 4.23: Semilobar holoprosencephaly: Single primitive ventricle (holoventricle) (arrow) seen with thalami (T) fused in the midline

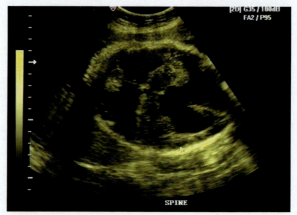

Fig. 4.24: Lobar holoprosencephaly: The septum pellucidum is absent but the inter-hemispheric fissure is well-developed posteriorly

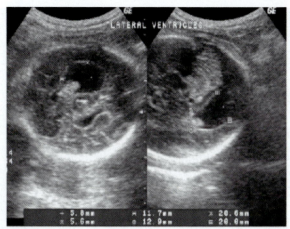

Fig. 4.25: Ventriculomegaly seen in the atrial and occipital regions (colpocephaly) because of poorly developed white matter surrounding these areas (Tear drop configuration) with an absent cavum septum pellucidum

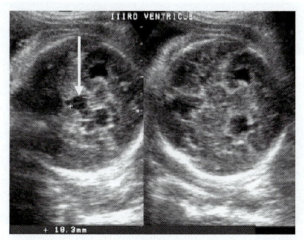

Fig. 4.26: An enlarged elevated third ventricle is seen between the hemispheres which appears as an inter-hemispheric cyst

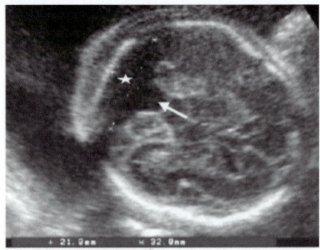

Fig. 4.27: Large cyst in the posterior cranial fossa (star) with a hypoplastic cerebellar vermis (arrow)

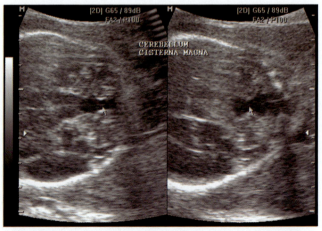

Fig. 4.28: Midline cyst in the posterior cranial fossa which is communicating (arrow) with the fourth ventricle

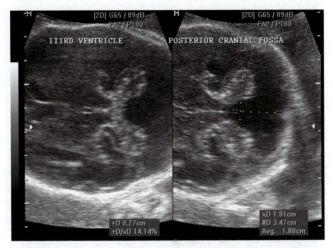

Fig. 4.29: Abnormally developed cerebellar vermis

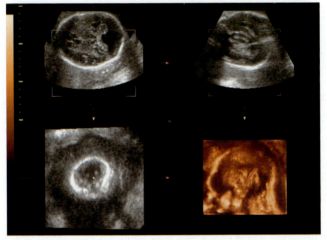

Fig. 4.30: DWM as seen on 3D with all planes visualized

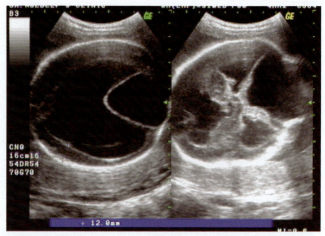

Fig. 4.31: Dandy-Walker malformation with hydrocephalus

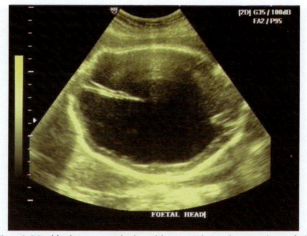

Fig. 4.32: Hydranencephaly with complete destruction of the cerebral cortex and basal ganglia with intact meninges and skull which is of normal appearance

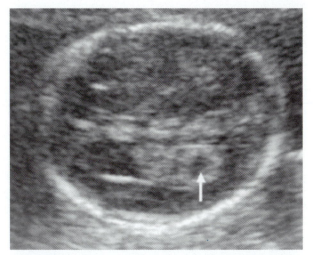

Fig. 4.33: Unilateral single (arrow) choroid plexus cyst

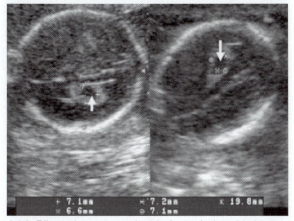

Fig. 4.34: Bilateral one on each side (arrow) choroid plexus cyst. A detailed scan to check for sonographic stigmata of chromosomal abnormalities especially Trisomy 18 is done and only if any additional anomaly is detected an amniocentesis is indicated for

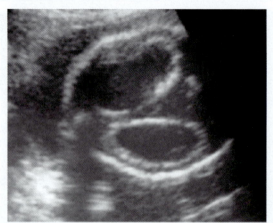

Fig. 4.35: Ventriculomegaly with hyperechoic walls and multiple foci of calcification seen in the brain substance

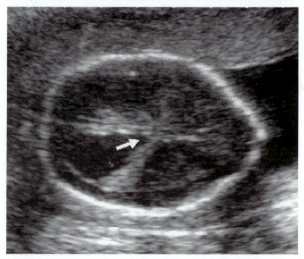

Fig. 4.36: Enlarged lateral ventricles with loss of the approximation between the choroid plexus and the medial border of the lateral ventricle (arrow)

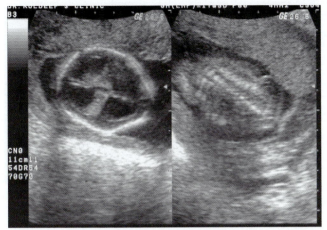

Fig. 4.37: Ventriculomegaly (left side) seen with a dysraphic disorganization of the lumbar and sacrococcygeal vertebrae

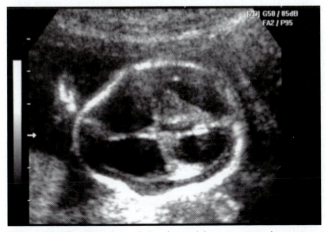

Fig. 4.38: Overlapping of the frontal bones seen in a case of communicating hydrocephalus

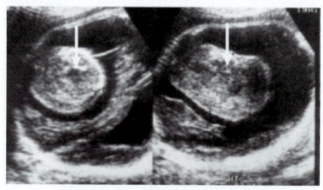

Fig. 4.39: Mass, possible a teratoma (arrows) with dilatation of the lateral ventricles

4.7 FETAL SPINE (FIGS 4.48 TO 4.59)

1. Coronal
2. Longitudinal
3. Axial ossification
4. Soft tissues.

4.8 FETAL THORAX (FIGS 4.60 TO 4.71)

1. Diaphragm
2. Lung length
3. Lung echoes
4. Ribs
5. Masses
6. Cardiothoracic ratio.

4.9 FETAL HEART (FIGS 4.72 TO 4.92)

1. Situs
2. Size
3. Rate

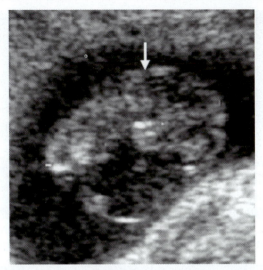

Fig. 4.40: Nuchal translucency in a 10 weeks fetus. Any thickening of the nuchal translucency prompts to a diagnosis of cystic hygroma, chromosomal abnormalities or cardiac abnormalities. Nuchal translucency in a 13 weeks fetus. Nuchal translucency thickness usually increases with gestational age with 1.5 mm and 2.5 mm being the 50th and 95th percentile respectively for gestational ages between 10 and 12 weeks. 2.0 mm and 3.0 mm are the 50th and 95th percentile respectively for gestational ages between 12 and 14 weeks

4. Rhythm
5. Configuration
6. Connections
7. Fetal circulation

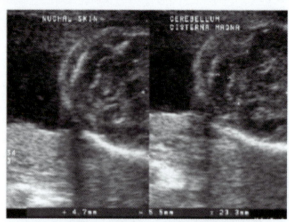

Fig. 4.41: Nuchal skin fold thickness assessment through the section for the cerebellum and cisterna magna

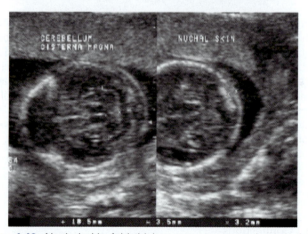

Fig. 4.42: Nuchal skin fold thickness assessment through the section just inferior to the section for cerebellum and cisterna magna. (14-18 weeks : Normal value < 4 mm, Borderline 4-5 mm and > 5 mm requires further karyotypic analysis) (18-22 weeks : Normal value < 5 mm, Borderline 5-6 mm and > 6 mm requires further karyotypic analysis)

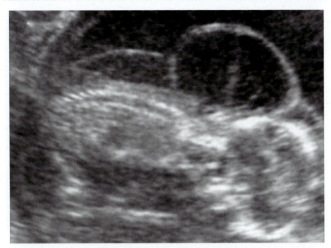

Fig. 4.43: Cystic hygroma seen in the longitudinal section across the entire fetal spine

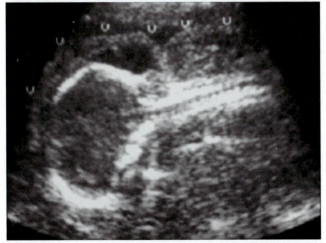

Fig. 4.44: Cystic hygroma seen in the longitudinal section posterior to the cranium, craniovertebral junction and cervical vertebra

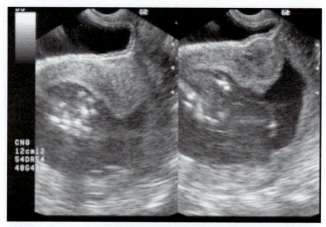

Fig. 4.45: Cystic hygroma seen as a diffuse lesion along the fetal thorax and abdomen

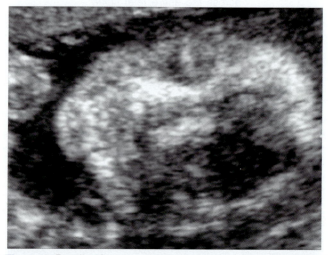

Fig. 4.46: Detailed facial anatomy which can be seen in a second trimester ultrasound. Note the eyelids, nose, lips, cheeks and chin which can be seen so clearly and can be shown to the expectant parents as well

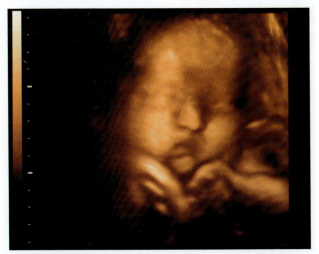

Fig. 4.47: Fetal face on 3 D reconstruction

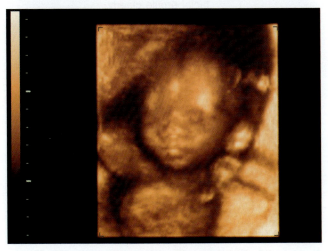

Fig. 4.48: Clear recognition of fetal facial
features as seen on 3D

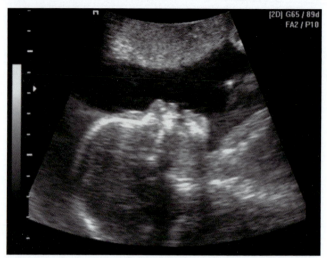

Fig. 4.49: Sagittal section through the mid-face showing the facial profile clearly

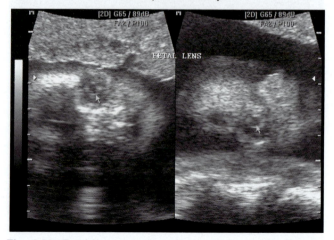

Fig. 4.50: Fetal lens seen in both the orbits on ultrasound is seen as a hyperechoic rim with a sonolucent center (arrow)

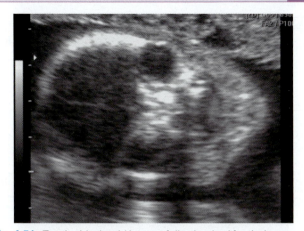

Fig. 4.51: Fetal orbit should be carefully checked for their osseous continuity apart from the measurements. View for the measurements of ocular diameter (measured from medial inner to medial lateral wall of the long orbit), interocular distance (measured from medial inner wall of one orbit to medial inner wall of the other orbit) and binocular distance (measured from lateral inner wall of one orbit to lateral inner wall of the other orbit)

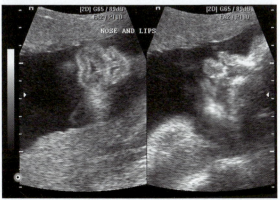

Fig. 4.52: Modified coronal view of the lower face showing the nostrils and the lips

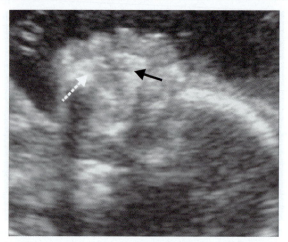

Fig. 4.53: Sagittal view showing the forehead, maxilla and mandible

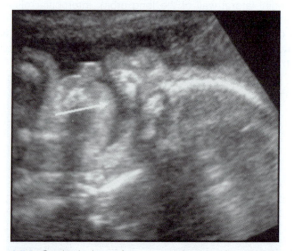

Fig. 4.54: Sagittal view of a normal fetal profile showing the osseous and soft tissue components. With the fetal mouth open the normal positioning of the tongue can also be seen

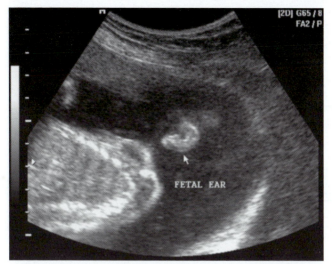

Fig. 4.55: Parasagittal view showing the external ear

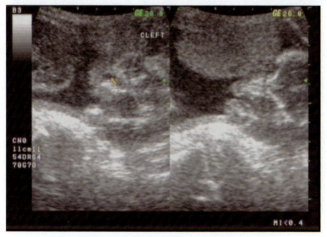

Fig. 4.56: Unilateral cleft lip extending into
the maxilla as well

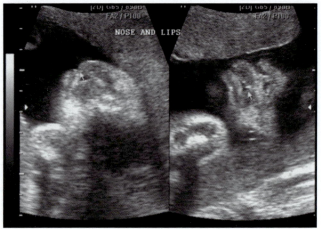

Fig. 4.57: Unilateral cleft lip (arrow). Note the dropout of echoes in the upper lip

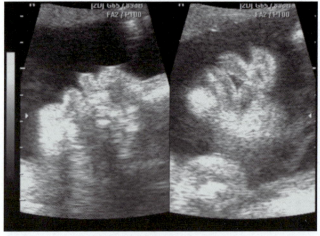

Fig. 4.58: Unilateral cleft lip

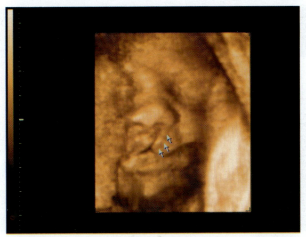

Fig. 4.59: 3D reconstruction of the cleft upper lip as shown on 2D in Figure 4.58. This helps the parents to understand better

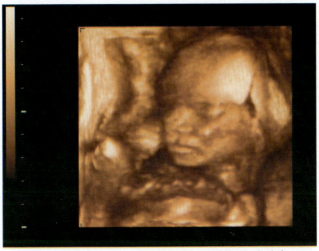

Fig. 4.60: 3D reconstruction of the bilateral cleft lip as seen from the side

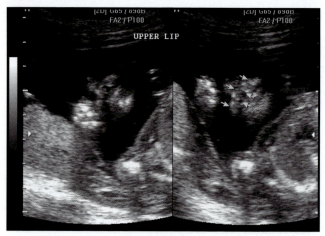

Fig. 4.61: Bilateral cleft lip and palate (arrows)

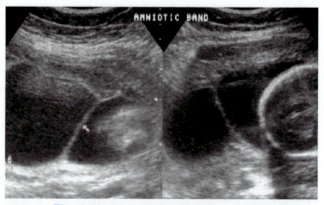

Fig. 4.62: Amniotic bands (arrow) can be associated with a cleft lip or palate

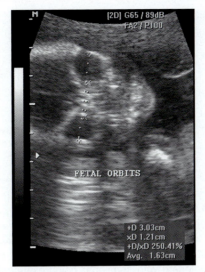

Fig. 4.63: Fetal orbits seen in the coronal view to assess for hypo/hypertelorism

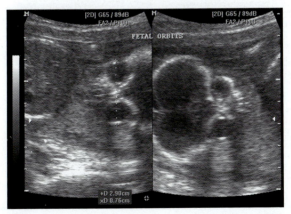

Fig. 4.64: Hypotelorism seen in a case of semilobar holoprosencephaly. The ocular diameter in this case was 12 mm, the interocular distance was 8 mm and the binocular distance was 29 mm

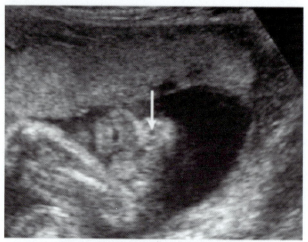

Fig. 4.65: Single nostril (arrow) seen in the case of hypotelorism with semilobar holoprosencephaly

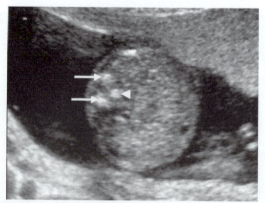

Fig. 4.66: Three ossification centers seen in the transverse plane. Two of these are posterior (arrows) and one is anterior (arrow head). Transverse planes to delineate any minimal widening of the interpedicular distance

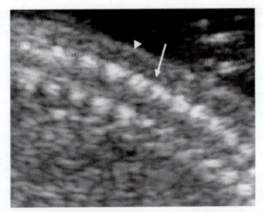

Fig. 4.67: The cutaneous, subcutaneous and muscular components seen posterior to the vertebral column all along the cervical,
dorsal, lumbar and sacrococcygeal vertebrae. The longitudinal
plane of the fetal spine delineating the soft tissues posterior to
the vertebral column and any dysraphic disorganization of the
spine

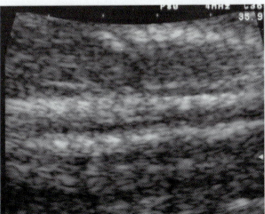

Fig. 4.68: Sagittal plane to delineate the spinal cord in the lower
cervical, dorsal and lumbar spine and to delineate any osseous
deformity

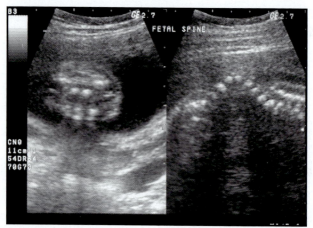

Fig. 4.69: Defect in the osseous component of the vertebral column and disruption of cutaneous and subcutaneous elements. Osseous disorganization of the fetal spine

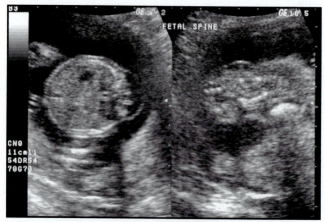

Fig. 4.70: Gross dysraphic disorganization of the entire spine

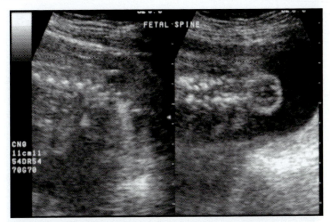

Fig. 4.71: Bulging membrane covering the vertebral lesion

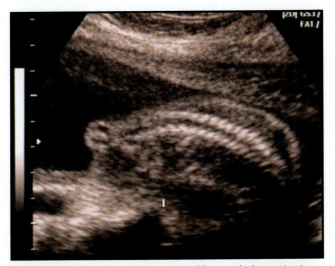

Fig. 4.72: Sacral meningocele with anechoic contents

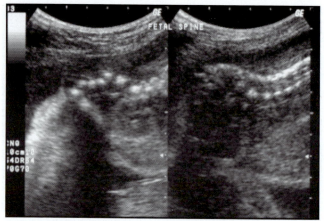

Fig. 4.73: Lumbosacral meningomyelocele

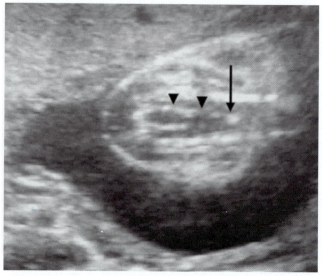

Fig. 4.74: Bony spicule (arrow) dividing the spinal cord
(arrow heads)

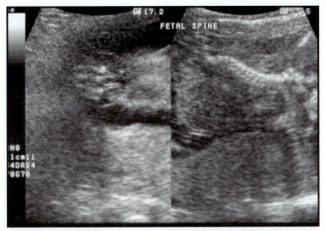

Fig. 4.75: Gross dysraphic disorganization of the entire fetal spine with a tethered spinal cord

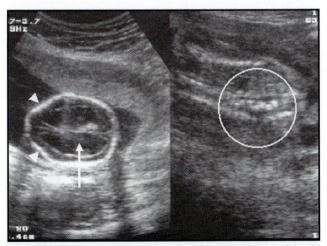

Fig. 4.76: Lumbosacral meningomyelocele (within circle) with associated dilatation of the lateral ventricles (arrow) and frontal bossing (lemon sign) (arrow heads)

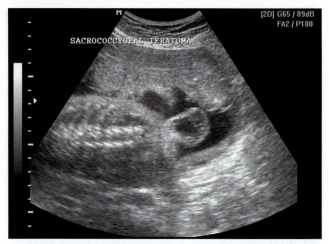

Fig. 4.77: Cystic sacrococcygeal teratoma

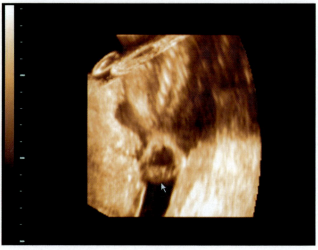

Fig. 4.78: 3D reconstruction of the postsacral mass

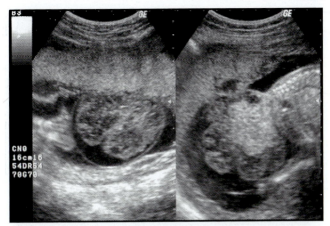

Fig. 4.79: Mass seen inferior to the sacrococcygeal area. Sacrococcygeal mass with a solid cum cystic echo pattern

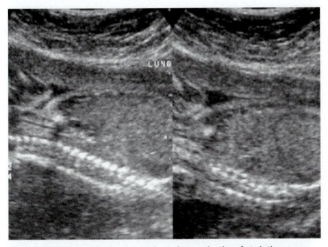

Fig. 4.80: Longitudinal section through the fetal thorax on both sides to assess the fetal lungs

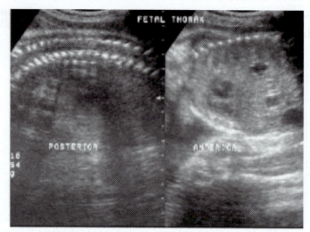

Fig. 4.81: Longitudinal section through the fetal thorax to assess the spine posteriorly (for osseous deformities, meningoceles or meningomyeloceles, anterior or posterior) and anterior thoracic wall anteriorly (for any thinning or ectopia cordis)

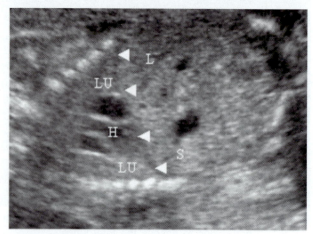

Fig. 4.82: Diffusely homogeneous fetal lung (LU) seen as diffuse low level echoes in comparison with the fetal liver (L). Diaphragm seen as arrow heads

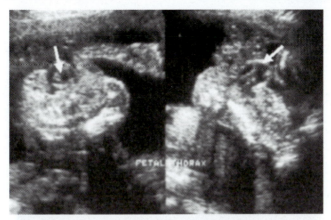

Fig. 4.83: Absent anterior thoracic wall with the fetal heart (arrow) seen outside the fetal thorax

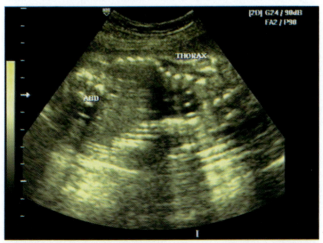

Fig. 4.84: Narrow fetal thorax in comparison with the fetal abdomen

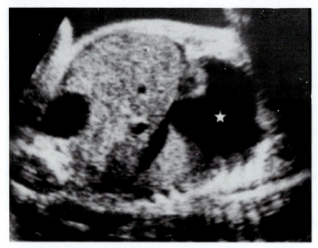

Fig. 4.85: Large pleural effusion (star) taking on the shape of the chest wall, diaphragm and mediastinal contour

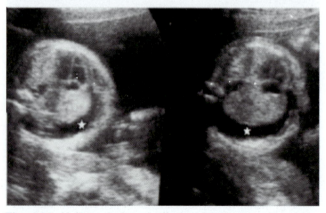

Fig. 4.86: Unilateral pleural effusion (star) taking the shape of the chest wall and mediastinum

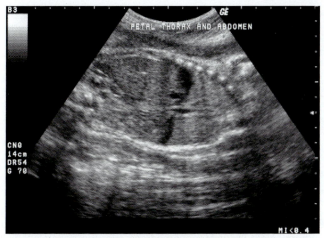

Fig. 4.87: Bilateral pleural effusion

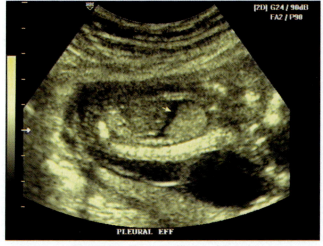

Fig. 4.88: Pleural effusion (arrow)

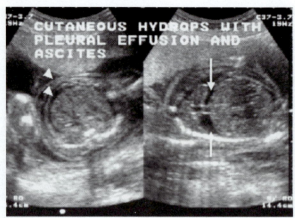

Fig. 4.89: Bilateral pleural effusion (arrow) as a part of generalised hydrops. Note the cutaneous hydrops over the abdominal wall and ascites

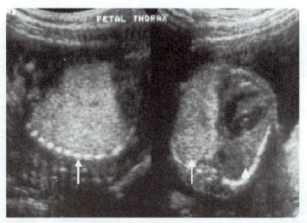

Fig. 4.90: Cystic adenomatoid malformation of the right lung (arrow). Because of distal acoustic enhancement from very small cysts the lesion appears as a solid mass. Note the difference in echo pattern from the left lung (arrow head)

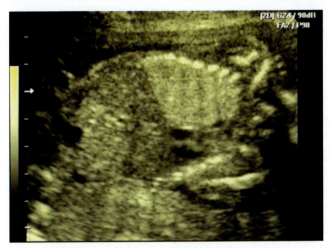

Fig. 4.91: Cystic adenomatoid malformation
of the fetal lung

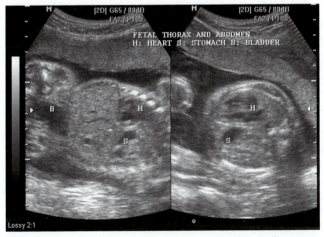

Fig. 4.92: Fetal stomach (S) seen in the retrocardiac area
with the diaphragm seen

4.10 FETAL ABDOMEN (FIGS 4.93 TO 4.168)

1. Gastrointestinal
   a. Stomach
   b. Duodenum
   c. Small bowel
   d. Large bowel
   e. Omentum
   f. Mesentery
2. Hepatobiliary
   a. Liver
   b. Gallbladder
3. Genitourinary
   a. Kidneys
   b. Ureters
   c. Urinary bladder
4. Pancreas
5. Spleen.

4.11 FETAL SKELETON

1. Cranium
2. Mandible
3. Clavicle
4. Spine
5. Extremities.

4.12 FETAL BIOMETRY

1. Biparietal diameter
2. Occipitofrontal distance
3. Head perimeter
4. Abdominal perimeter
5. Femoral length
6. Humeral length.

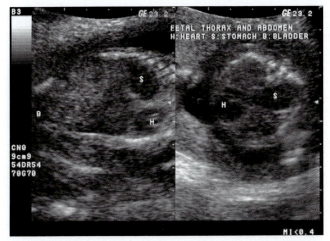

Fig. 4.93: Fetal stomach seen posterior to the fetal heart as seen in a longitudinal and transverse section

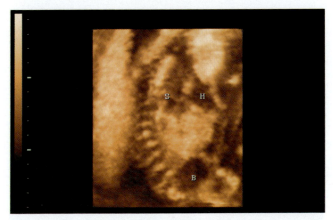

Fig. 4.94: Congenital diaphragmatic hernia as seen on 3D

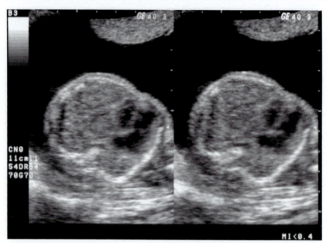

Fig. 4.95: Right sided diaphragmatic hernia. The mass is almost isoechoic with the lung

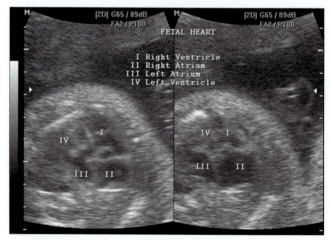

Fig. 4.96: Cardiac four-chamber view. Please note that with the spine lateral or posterior one can get a good four chamber view of the heart

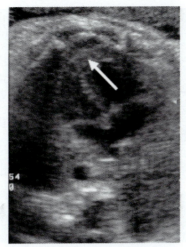

Fig. 4.97: Moderator band (arrow) seen in the right ventricle at the apex

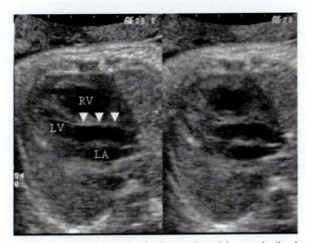

Fig. 4.98: Aortoseptal continuity (arrow heads) seen in the long axis view. The left ventricle (LV), right ventricle (RV) and left atrium (LA) are also labeled

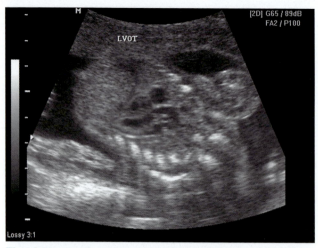

Fig. 4.99: Another view of the left ventricular outflow tract showing aortoseptal continuity

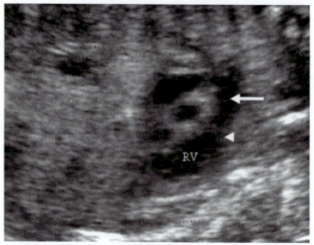

Fig. 4.100: Right ventricle (RV), pulmonary valve (arrow head) and pulmonary artery (arrow) seen as the right ventricular outflow tract

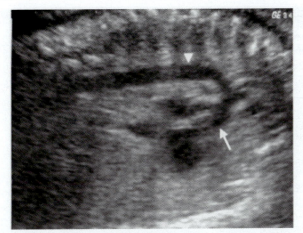

Fig. 4.101: Right ventricular outflow tract with the pulmonary artery (arrow) from the right ventricle going into the ductus arteriosus and descending aorta (arrow head)

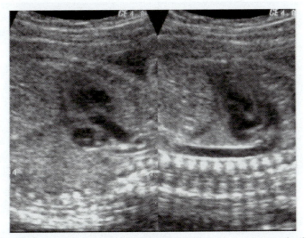

Fig. 4.102: Left ventricular outflow tract with aortoseptal continuity (left side) and right ventricular outflow tract with the pulmonary artery (right side) shown

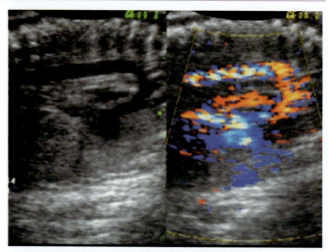

Fig. 4.103: Aortic arch seen from the fetal heart and its branches in the neck

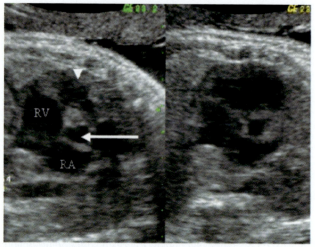

Fig. 4.104: Right atrium (RA), right ventricle (RV) and pulmonary artery (arrow head) seen in the short axis view encircling the aorta (arrow)

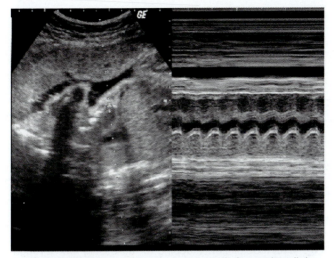

Fig. 4.105: M-mode tracings to check for pericardial effusion, chamber size and wall thickness

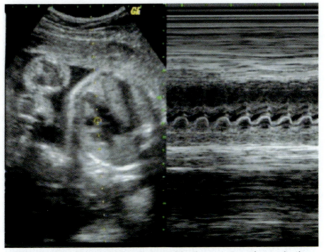

Fig. 4.106: M-mode tracings with the cursor through the right ventricle, left ventricle and left atrium

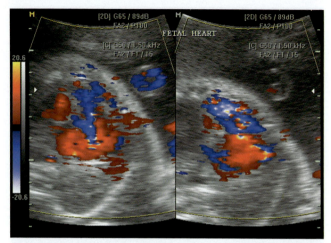

Fig. 4.107: Color flow mapping for assessing flow through the atrioventricular valves

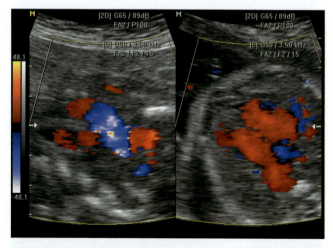

Fig. 4.108: Color flow mapping for assessing flow through and distal to the semilunar valves

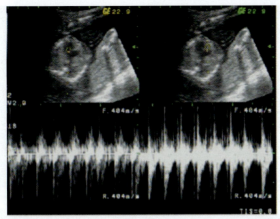

Fig. 4.109: Doppler gate for sampling for arterial flow velocities across the atrioventricular valves for peak flow velocities and volume flow across these valves for delineation of stenosis or regurgitation

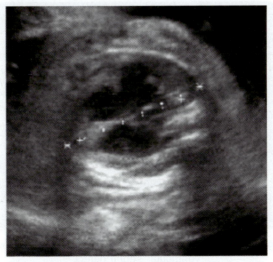

Fig. 4.110: Cardiomegaly with the cardiothoracic ratio in this case as 80%

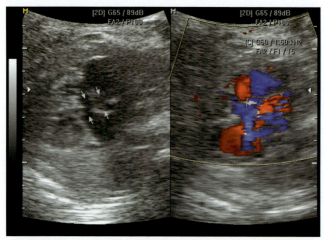

Fig. 4.111: Four chamber view with a large ventricular septal defect (arrows) and an atrial septal defect

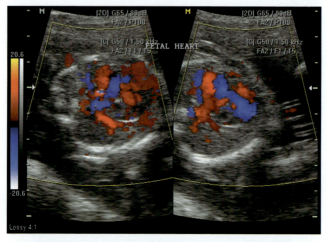

Fig. 4.112: Four chamber view with a perimembranous ventricular septal defect

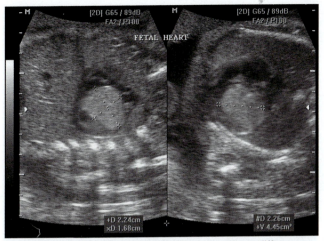

Fig. 4.113: Cardiac rhabdomyoma with a diffuse thickening of the myocardium

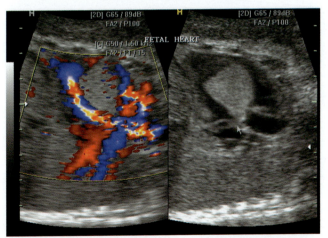

Fig. 4.114: Outflow tracts seen on color flow mapping around the rhabdomyoma

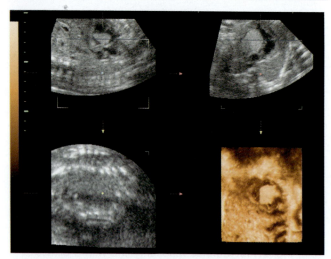

Fig. 4.115: Cardiac tumor as seen on 3D

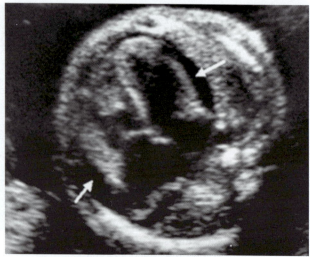

Fig. 4.116: Pericardial effusion (arrow) seen
enveloping the fetal heart

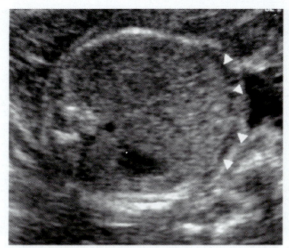

Fig. 4.117: Pseudoascites (arrow heads) is the hypoechoic area seen only along the anterior and lateral aspects on the periphery commonly seen in a transverse section

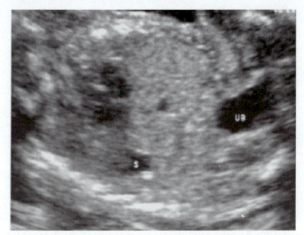

Fig. 4.118: Fluid filled structures, stomach (S) and urinary bladder (UB) seen in the fetal abdomen

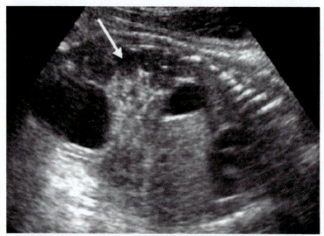

Fig. 4.119: Normal colonic echoes (hypoechoic) seen at the periphery of the fetal abdomen (arrow)

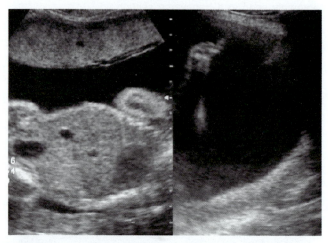

Fig. 4.120: Esophageal atresia as diagnosed by demonstration of polyhydramnios (right side) with an inability to visualize the stomach bubble (left side)

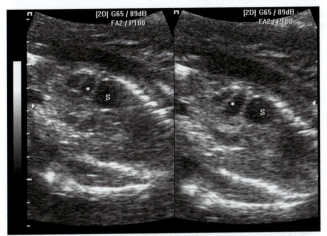

Fig. 4.121: Double bubble sign seen as a distended stomach (S) and an enlarged duodenal bulb (star)

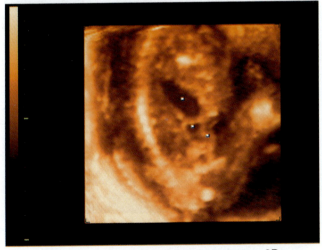

Fig. 4.122: Duodenal atresia as seen on 3D

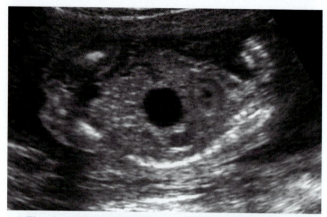

Fig. 4.123: Duodenal atresia with fetal stomach and duodenal bulb

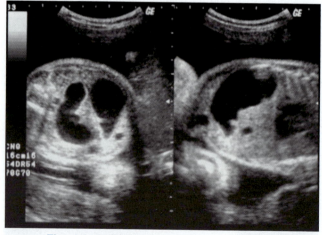

Fig. 4.124: Dilated stomach and duodenum

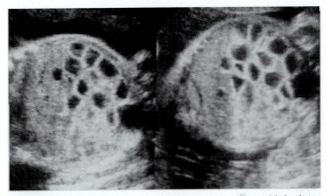

Fig. 4.125: Small bowel obstruction seen as multiple inter-connecting, overdistended bowel loops more than 7 mm in diameter. Take care that you do not confuse the same picture with a multicystic dysplastic kidney or a dilated tortuous ureter

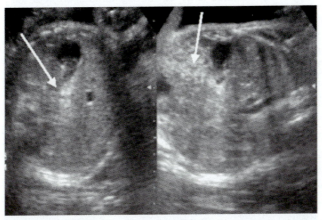

Fig. 4.126: Echogenic bowel (arrow) which can be normally seen in a normal fetus at term with hyperechoic colonic meconium or hyperechoic bowel contents in the fetus who has swallowed intra-amniotic blood

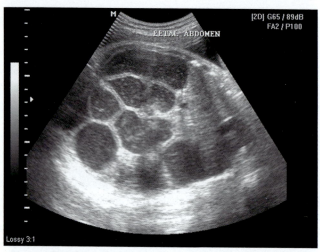

Fig. 4.127: Dilated large bowel segments seen near the periphery in a case of anorectal malformation

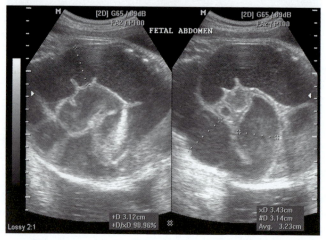

Fig. 4.128: Dilated large bowel loops (30-34 mm)

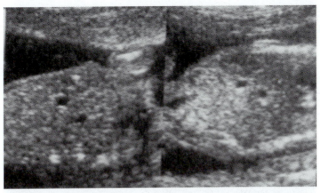

Fig. 4.129: Scattered echogenic foci with distal acoustic shadowing in a case of meconium peritonitis

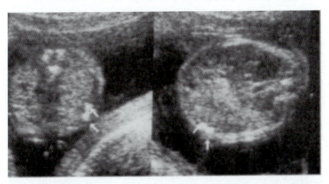

Fig. 4.130: Dense hyperechoic foci (arrows) seen in the periphery in a case of meconium peritonitis

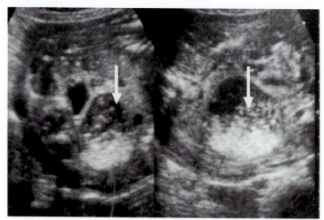

Fig. 4.131: Meconium peritonitis with a meconium pseudocyst (arrow) with debris seen within it

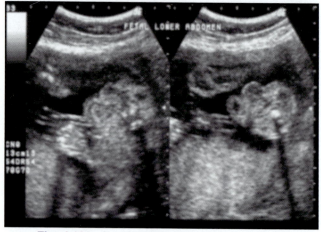

Fig. 4.132: Gastroschisis with bowel segments seen floating freely in the amniotic fluid

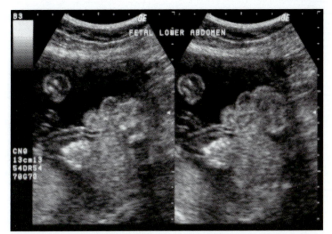

Fig. 4.133: Gastroschisis with bowel loops floating and on 2 D ultrasound the umbilical cord is seen on the side of the lesion

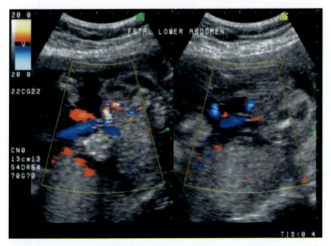

Fig. 4.134: Anterior abdominal wall defect (gastroschisis) with the umbilical cord insertion on the side of the lesion as seen on color flow mapping

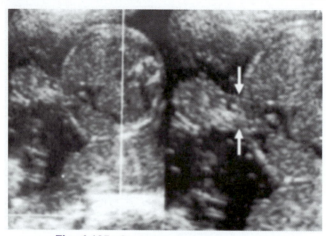

Fig. 4.135: Omphalocele (arrow) seen in a case of trisomy 18

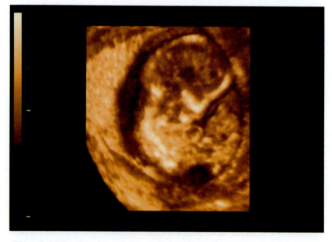

Fig. 4.136: Omphalocele with abdominal viscera herniating as seen on 3D

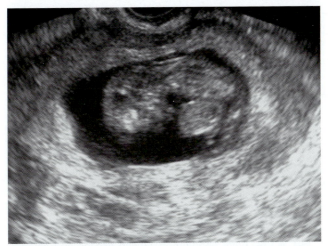

Fig. 4.137: Omphalocele in an early second trimester fetus

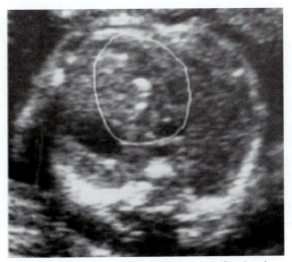

Fig. 4.138: Multiple foci of hepatic calcification in a case of intrauterine infection

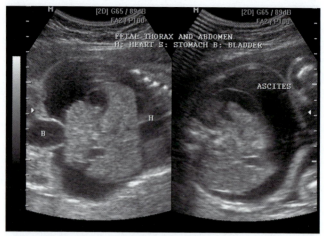

Fig. 4.139: Fetal hepatomegaly with ascites and ascites seen in a case of toxoplasmosis infection

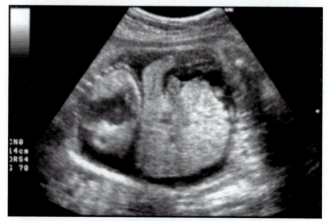

Fig. 4.140: Fetal hepatomegaly with gross fetal ascites seen in a case of severe fetal hydrops

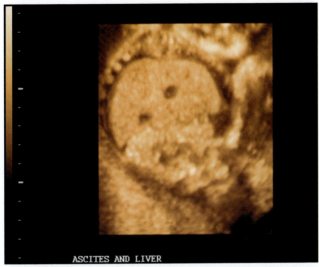

ASCITES AND LIVER

Fig. 4.141: Fetal hepatomegaly and ascites as seen on 3D

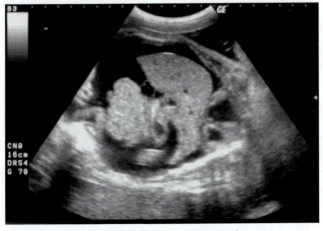

Fig. 4.142: Fetal hepatomegaly

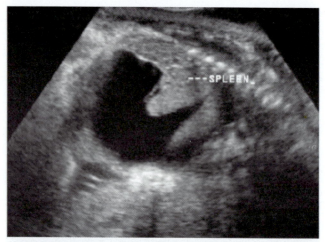

Fig. 4.143: Fetal splenomegaly (labeled) in a case of severe fetal hydrops

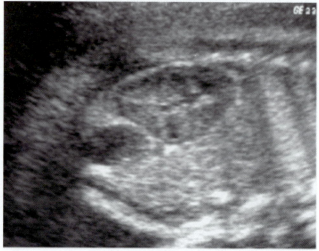

Fig. 4.144: Longitudinal scan of a normal kidney with its characteristic reniform shape

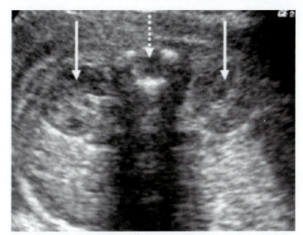

Fig. 4.145: Transverse section through the fetal abdomen showing both kidneys (arrow) on either side of the spine (dashed arrow)

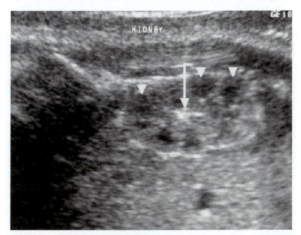

Fig. 4.146: Longitudinal scan of a normal kidney in the third trimester in a fetus of 33 weeks and 4 days. Note the central echogenic area (arrow) with hypoechoic pyramids (arrow heads)

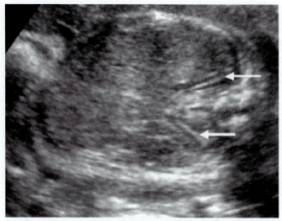

Fig. 4.147: Fetal adrenal glands as seen normally (arrow). Be careful not to mistake the adrenal for a kidney especially in cases of renal agenesis. To differentiate remember that the adrenal gland does not have central sinus echoes and a reniform shape

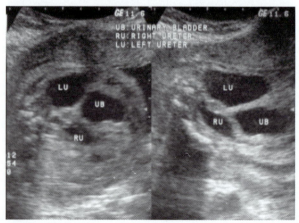

Fig. 4.148: Obstruction of the urinary tract at the bladder outlet with an overdistended urinary bladder, dilated ureters on both sides and a bilateral hydronephrosis

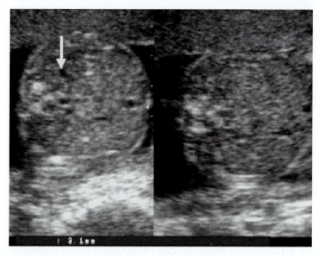

Fig. 4.149: Anteroposterior diameter of the renal pelvis (arrow). The values for the anteroposterior diameter of the renal pelvis (measured on a transverse view through the kidney) are from 15 to 20 weeks of gestation < 4 mm is normal, 4 to 7 mm is borderline and > 8 mm is abnormal or hydronephrotic. From 20 weeks onwards < 6 mm is normal, 6 to 9 is borderline and > 10 mm is abnormal or hydronephrotic. Be careful that borderline cases are to be reviewed by serial scans before labeling them as hydronephrotic

4.13 EXTRA-FETAL EVALUATION

1. Placenta (Location, morphology, focal lesions, retroplacental area) (Figs 4.169 to 4.173)
2. Liquor amnii (Normal, oligohydramnios, polyhydramnios, amniotic bands) (Figs 4.174 to 4.177)
3. Umbilical cord (Number of Vessels, Origin and Insertion, Masses) (Figs 4.178 to 4.182)

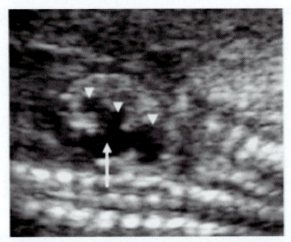

Fig. 4.150: Pelvi-ureteric junction obstruction with a dilated renal pelvis (arrow) with dilated calyces (arrow heads) No ureteric dilatation is seen

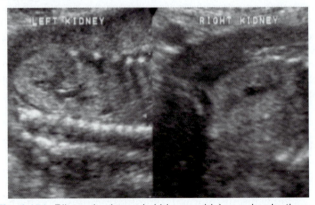

Fig. 4.151: Bilateral echogenic kidneys which are dysplastic and small with very less pelviectasis. This is not a reduction in hydronephrosis as the improvement with dysplastic kidney is because the renal function is poor or absent and is not going to improve even after the obstruction is corrected

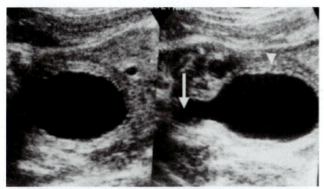

Fig. 4.152: Bladder outlet obstruction with dilatation of the proximal urethra (arrow) and a thickened urinary bladder wall (arrow head)

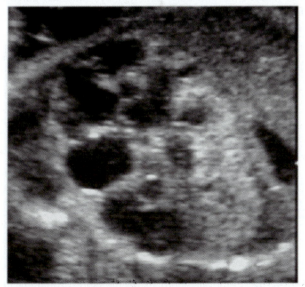

Fig. 4.153: Multicystic dysplastic kidney with multiple cysts and no normal renal parenchyma seen

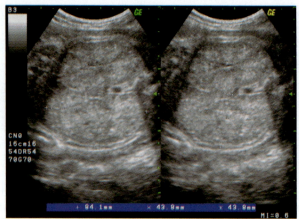

Fig. 4.154: Enlarged echogenic kidneys (infantile polycystic kidney disease) with severe oligohydramnios and non-visualization of the urinary bladder

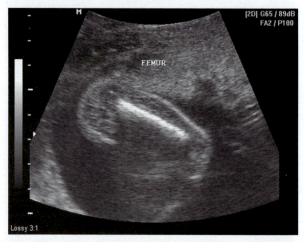

Fig. 4.155: Femoral length to be measured routinely in all obstetric ultrasound after 14 weeks. If a skeletal deformity is being suspected the tibial and fibular lengths also to be taken

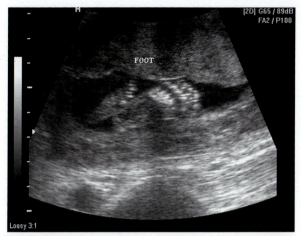

Fig. 4.156: Fetal feet to be checked for their orientation with the tibia to make a diagnosis of club foot

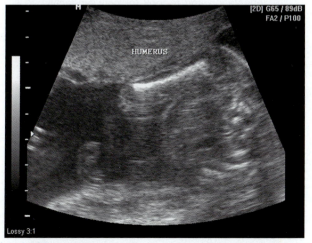

Fig. 4.157: Humeral length to be measured in all anomaly targeted obstetric ultrasound especially for chromosomal abnormalities after 14 weeks. If a skeletal deformity is being suspected the radial and ulnar lengths also to be taken

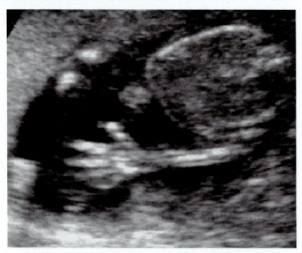

Fig. 4.158: Fetal hands to be checked for position, orientation and to look for poly/syndactyly

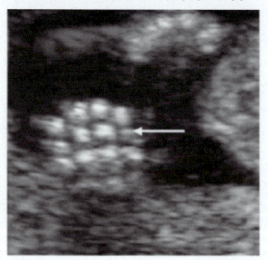

Fig. 4.159: The fifth digit should be carefully assessed for any incurving or any hypoplasia of the middle phalanx of the fifth digit (arrow)

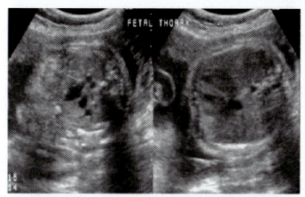

Fig. 4.160: Narrowing of the fetal thorax to be assessed by taking the thoracic perimeter and checking the abdominal perimeter/ thoracic perimeter ratio. One should also assess by taking the maximium antero-posterior measurement of the thorax and the abdomen on a longitudinal section. Configuration of ribs to be seen on both sides to check for any thoracic narrowing with resultant pulmonary hypoplasia and a bad prognosis

```
         MEAN( mm, mm² ) GA
BPD(CAM)  47.6    19w5d ±1w0d
OFD(HAN)  58.3    19w4d ±5.30mm
HC (HAD) 164.1    19w1d ±1w3d
AC (HAD) 137.5    19w1d ±2w0d
FL (HAD)  20.3    16w0d ±1w3d
HUM(JEA)  20.3    16w0d ±2w5d
RAD(MEZ)  13.9    15w3d ±3.50mm
ULN(JEA)  15.2    15w1d ±3w0d
TIB(JEA)  13.5    14w4d ±2w6d
FIB(MEZ)  12.8    14w3d ±3.00mm
THD(HAN)  32.0    16w0d ±4.70mm
```

Fig. 4.161: Report on parameters of a case of thanatophoric dysplasia. Cranial parameters and abdominal perimeter correspond to 19-20 weeks size, thoracic dimensions to 16 weeks size and bone lengths to 14-15 weeks size

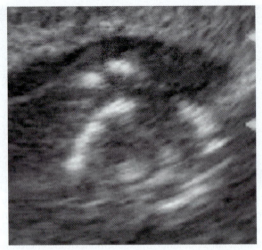

Fig. 4.162: Bowed long bones almost giving a telephone receiver appearance

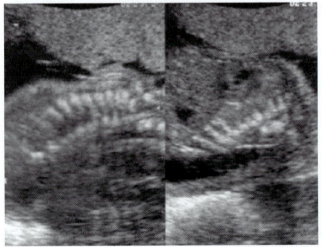

Fig. 4.163: Narrow thorax, in the longitudinal section compare the side to side measurement of the fetal thorax and abdomen

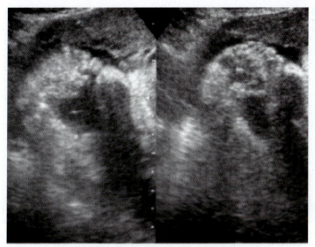

Fig. 4.164: Fetal foot turned medially in a case of club foot

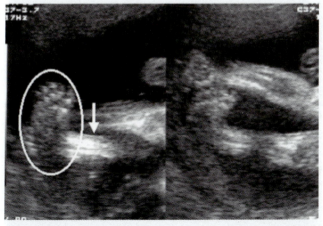

Fig. 4.165: Visualize the sole of the foot (within circle) and if in this view you can see the tibia (arrow) it is a club foot deformity

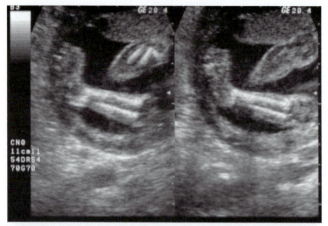

Fig. 4.166: Clubfoot deformity can be associated with Trisomy 18, so a thorough check for stigmata of Trisomy 18 should be done

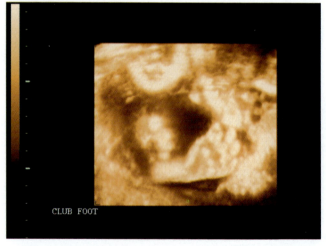

Fig. 4.167: Clubfoot as seen on 3 D reconstruction

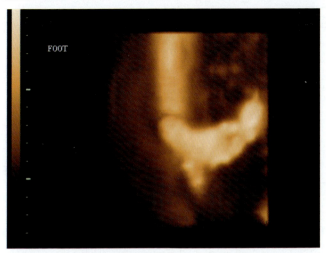

Fig. 4.168: 3D view of clubfoot

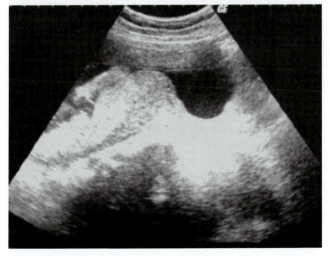

Fig. 4.169: An upper segment placenta as the placenta in this case is far away from the internal os

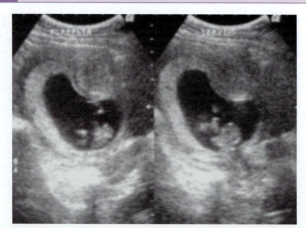

Fig. 4.170: The placenta is posterior. Its inferior limit extends down to the internal os but does not span across it

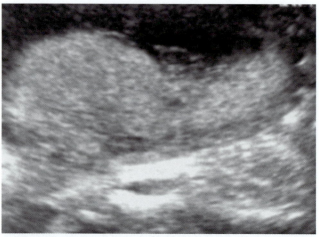

Fig. 4.171: Grade I placenta at 20 weeks and 2 days

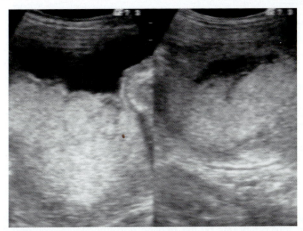

Fig. 4.172: Multiple anechoic or hypoechoic areas near the fetal surface or the uterine surface of the placenta are seen. The only focal lesion of significance is chorioangioma which is hypoechoic and very vascular

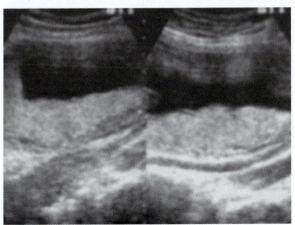

Fig. 4.173: The retroplacental area usually appears hypoechoic because of vessels, so do not mistake it as retroplacental collection

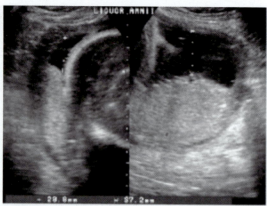

Fig. 4.174: Amniotic fluid index assessment. The uterus is divided into four quadrants by the midline and transverse axis and the amniotic fluid as the deepest vertical pocket free of fetal parts and umbilical cord is measured in each quadrant and all four quadrants add up to give the amniotic fluid index. Gradation of the amniotic fluid into oligo/polyhydramnios is then done

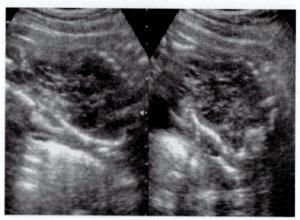

Fig. 4.175: Severe oligohydramnios in a case of bilateral renal agenesis. Note the complete absence of liquor amnii with the uterine wall closely apposed to the fetus

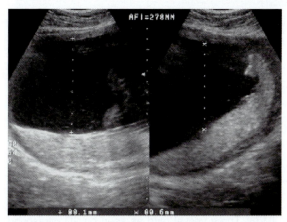

Fig. 4.176: Moderate polyhydramnios in a case of congenital diaphragmatic hernia. Diagnosis is striking in these cases as the fetus is seen freely mobile in liquor amnii. Both pockets shown in the picture are more than 80 mm each

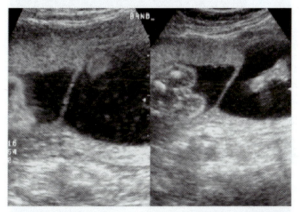

Fig. 4.177: Amniotic fold/band seen traversing the uterine cavity. Be careful to check for any limb or digit reduction/constriction defects, external anomalies of the face (cleft lip and palate, nasal abnormalities), cranum (anencephaly or encephalocele), anterior abdominal wall defects and abnormal curvature of the spine

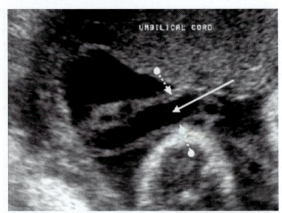

Fig. 4.178: Three vessel cord as seen on 2D ultrasound. The single umbilical vein (arrow) and two umbilical arteries (dotted arrows) are seen as a rail track appearance

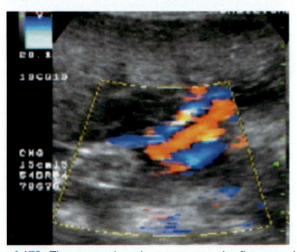

Fig. 4.179: Three vessel cord as seen on color flow mapping. Two umbilical arteries (blue) and single umbilical vein (red) can be easily demonstrated. On color flow mapping the red and blue to not specify arteries and veins but flow towards the transducer or away from it

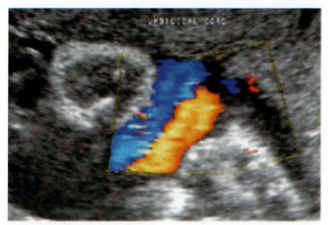

Fig. 4.180: Two vessel cord as seen on color flow mapping. Single umbilical artery and single umbilical vein can be seen

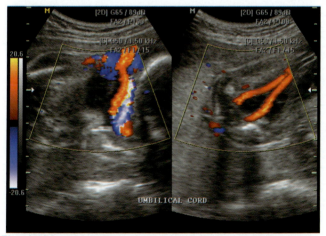

Fig. 4.181: Hypogastric arteries seen adjacent to the urinary bladder on both sides confirming a three vessel cord

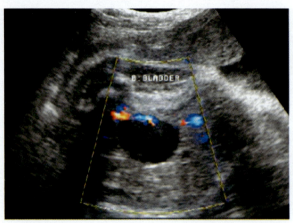

Fig. 4.182: Hypogastric artery seen adjacent to the urinary bladder only on one side confirming a two vessel cord seen in Figure 4.181

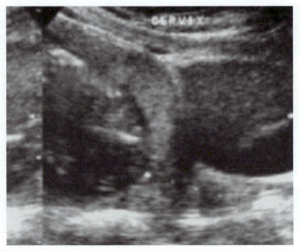

Fig. 4.183: The internal os should be seen whether it is open or not and whether there is any herniation as well

4. Cervix (Internal os width, Length of cervix and Serial evaluation) (Figs 4.183 to 4.185)
5. Lower segment (Thickness)
6. Myometrium (Masses) (Fig. 4.186)
7. Adnexa (Masses) (Fig. 4.187).

4.14 COLOR DOPPLER IN SECOND TRIMESTER

1. Uterine artery
2. Umbilical artery
3. Fetal circulation
4. Placental perfusion.

4.15 3D AND 4D SCAN

1. Surface anatomy
2. Anomaly scan
3. Bone and spine evaluation
4. 4D scan for maternal-fetal and family-fetal bonding

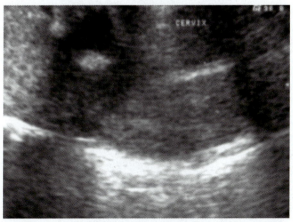

Fig. 4.184: Length: The cervical length is measured from the internal os to the external os or the mucus plug is measured

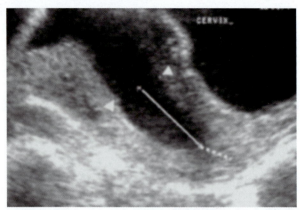

Fig. 4.185: Patient of cervical incompetence. The internal os (arrow heads) is open and 18 mm wide. The herniation of the amnion in the cervical canal (line) is over a distance of 32 mm. The functional or closed cervix (dashed line) which is required for the cerclage is 13 mm long

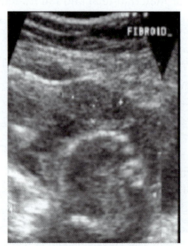

Fig. 4.186: An anterior wall subserous fibroid in a 16 weeks pregnancy

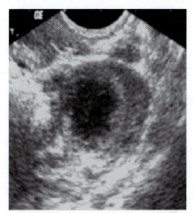

Fig. 4.187: Persistent corpus luteum in a 19 weeks pregnancy

4.16 ABNORMAL SECOND TRIMESTER

1. Low placenta
2. Separation
3. Oligo/polyhydramnios
4. Single umbilical artery
5. Incompetent os
6. Short cervix
7. Malformations.

4.17 DILEMMAS

1. Is it that with ultrasound one can find out each and every problem with the fetus, color Doppler is even better and is 3D the ultimate
2. Which period is best for diagnosing anomalies
3. Is the baby low
4. Will water drinking help for making of liquor
5. Ultrasound done at 13 weeks was normal, let's skip this scan.

Third Trimester

5.1 INDICATIONS

1. Suspected abruptio placentae
2. Estimation of fetal weight and/or presentation in premature rupture of membranes and/or premature labor
3. Serial evaluation of fetal growth in multiple gestations
4. Estimation of gestational age in late registrants for prenatal care

5. Biophysical profile for fetal well-being
6. Determination of fetal presentation
7. Suspected fetal death
8. Observation of intrapartum events
9. Suspected polyhydramnios or oligohydramnios.

5.2 FETAL EVALUATION

1. *Presentation:* Cephalic/breech(Extended or footling)/ oblique (Cranium in iliac fossae or hypochondrium (Figs 5.1 and 5.2).
2. Movements and biophysical score
3. Viability
4. *Gestational age:* Denotes fetal maturity (Fig. 5.3).
5. *Biometry:* Denotes fetal size and weight (Figs 5.4 to 5.6)
6. Color Doppler for fetal well-being

5.3 EXTRA-FETAL EVALUATION

1. *Placenta:* Grade I/II (with basal stippling)/III (with calcification) (Figs 5.7 and 5.8)
2. *Liquor amnii:* Normal/oligohydramnios/poly- hydramnios (Figs 5.9 to 5.11)
3. *Umbilical cord:* Presenting/around neck (Figs 5.12 to 5.14)
4. *Cervix:* Effaced/uneffaced
5. *Lower segment:* Thick (normorange)/thinned (Fig. 5.15)
6. Myometrium
7. Adnexa.

5.4 PLACENTAL CHECKLIST

1. Site of placentation
2. Relation of lower pole to internal os < 3 cm placenta previa > 3 cm-5 low lying > 5 cm away normal placentation site

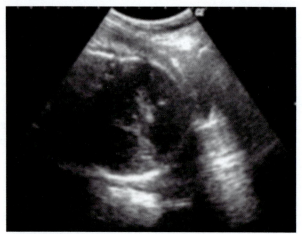

Fig. 5.1: Cephalic presentation with the cranium opposed to the cervix

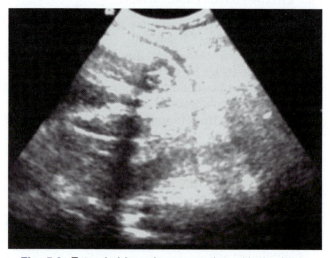

Fig. 5.2: Extended breech presentation with the fetal buttocks opposed to the cervix

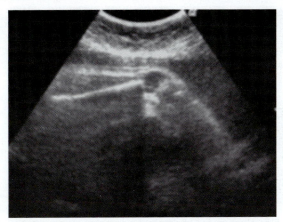

Fig. 5.3: The distal femoral epiphysis can be measured and maturity known as it starts appearing only after 35 weeks

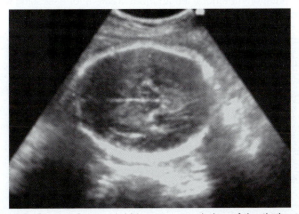

Fig. 5.4: Section for cranial biometry consisting of the thalamus, the third ventricle and the cavum septum pellucidum. The biparietal diameter is the side to side measurement from the outer table of the proximal skull to the inner table of the distal skull. The head perimeter is the total cranial circumference, which includes the maximum anteroposterior diameter. The occipitofrontal diameter is the front to back measurement from the outer table on both sides

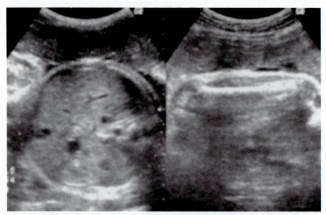

Fig. 5.5: Section for abdominal perimeter measurement. The spine should be posterior and the umbilical part of the portal vein anteriorly. Femoral length measurement for assessing fetal biometry

```
LMP(OPE)23/11/02  GA(LMP)34W0D EDD(LMP)30/08/03  GO PO AO EO
Ref MD:                    NOTE:
           POS:                PLAC:                        ← 1/2 ■
MEASUREMENTS CUA  LAST       1     2    3        AGE           GP
BPD(HADLOCK)  y   84.6mm  ( 84.6                ) 34W0D±3W1D 50%
HC(HADLOCK)   y   309mm   ( 309                 ) 34W4D±3W0D 26%
OFD(HC)           112mm   ( 112                 )
AC(HADLOCK)   y   296mm   ( 296                 ) 33W4D±3W0D 40%
FL(HADLOCK)   y   67.4mm  ( 67.4                ) 34W5D±3W0D 50%
CRL(HADLOCK)  y           (                     )
GS(HELLMAN)   y           (                     )




 CALCULATIONS
CI      75.7(70-86)           EFW 2328g±349g ( 5lb  2oz)  44%
FL/BPD  79.7(71-87)           Based On:(BPD HC AC  FL      )
FL/AC   22.8(20-24)           AFI(cm)           HR(BPM)
FL/HC   21.8(19.4-21.8)       LMP:(OPE)29/11/02
HC/AC   1.046(0.95-1.11)      AGE: LMP 34W0D    CUA 34W0D
                              EDD: LMP 30/08/03 CUA 30/08/03
COMMENTS:
```

Fig. 5.6: The chart shows a fetal weight of 2328 grams for 34 weeks with an EDD of 30/08/03

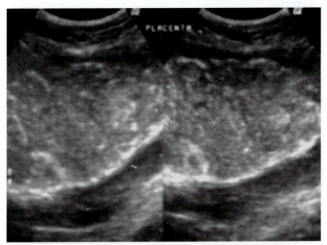

Fig. 5.7: Grade II placenta with basal stippling

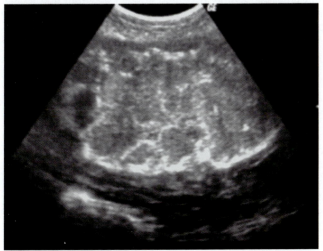

Fig. 5.8: Grade III placenta with calcification along the
basal plate, chorionic plate and intercotyledons

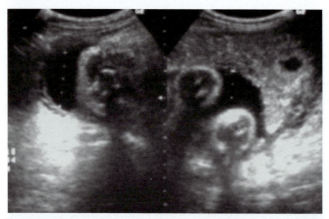

Fig. 5.9: Amniotic fluid index assessment. The uterus is divided into four quadrants by the midline and transverse axis and the amniotic fluid as the deepest vertical pocket free of fetal parts and umbilical cord is measured in each quadrant and all four quadrants add up to give the amniotic fluid index. Pregnancy of 38 weeks and 5 days with normal liquor amnii

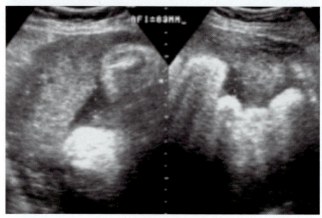

Fig. 5.10: Pregnancy of 37 weeks and 2 days with oligohydramnios

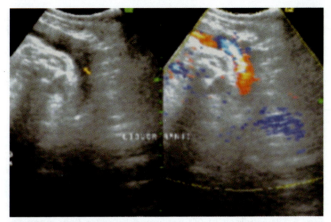

Fig. 5.11: Remember that if you have a color Doppler switch on the color to measure the pocket of liquor because many a times there is only cord in that pocket and it will give a wrong amniotic fluid index. Pocket which is full of umbilical cord so this pocket measurement is 0 mm not 28 mm as originally thought on a 2D image

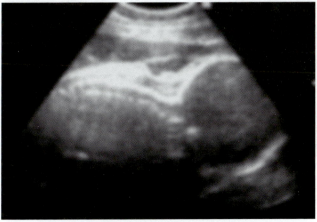

Fig. 5.12: Strong suspicion of two loops of umbilical cord on a 2D image

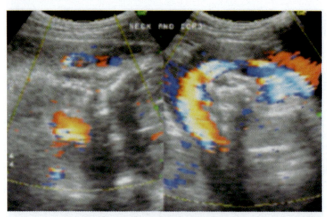

Fig. 5.13: Findings of 2D confirmed by color flow mapping when these two loops are demonstrated

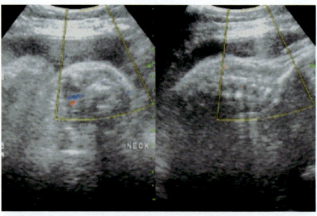

Fig. 5.14: No cord seen near or around the fetal neck as seen on color flow mapping

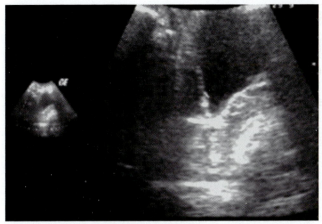

Fig. 5.15: Thinned lower segment scar seen in a patient of previous cesarean

3. Grading for maturity (immature, mature or hypermature) only hypermature placenta before 34 weeks gestation is of significance
4. Check for hypoechoic since in between placenta and uterine wall (rules out placenta acreta)
5. Check for retroplacental clot, abruptions, intraplacental hematomas, calcification
6. Color flow imaging (angio) for number of placental vessels and vasculature (to rule out placental insufficiency and infact).

5.5 AMNIOTIC FLUID ASSESSMENT

Condition	Single pocket	AFI
Oligohydramnios	< 2 cm	< 7
Reduced	2-3 cm	7-10
Normal	3-8 cm	10-17
More than average	> 8-12	17-25
Polyhydramnios	> 12	> 25

Scan whole uterine cavity for single pocket measure largest vertical pool for AFI four quadrant method.

5.6 CAUSES OF OLIGOHYDRAMNIOS

1. Idiopathic
2. Decreased urine production because of bilateral renal disease (primarily renal/secondary renal dysfunction)
3. Post-compensatory sequelae of intrauterine growth retardation.
4. Rupture of membranes
5. Postmaturity.

5.7 CAUSES OF POLYHYDRAMNIOS

1. Idiopathic
2. Open neural tube defects, e.g. encephalocele, meningo-myelocele, anencephaly.
3. Abnormalities primarily due to gastrointestinal obstruction, e.g. esophageal atresia, duodenal atresia, small bowel atresia/ obstruction or secondarily due to compression of the gastrointestinal system, e.g. cystic adenomatoid malformation, mass in the mediastinum, diaphragmatic hernia commonly left side.

4. Maternal diabetes mellitus
5. Fetal hydrops (immune or non-immune)
6. Chromosomal abnormality: Trisomy 18.

5.8 FETAL GROWTH

Fetal growth scan influenced by:
1. Small
2. Large
3. PIH
4. APH
5. Medical disorder in pregnancy
6. PROM
7. H/O previous small births.

IUGR/FGR

Causes
1. Low growth potential (Intrinsic factors)
   a. Genetic predisposition
   b. Chromosomal anomaly
   c. Fetal infection
   d. Structural fetal defects
   e. Drugs and medications.
2. Loss of growth support (Extrinsic factors)
   a. Unknown cause
   b. PIH
   c. Diabetes
   d. Lupus
   e. Recurrent bleeding episodes
   f. Multiple pregnancy
   g. Malnutrition
   h. Drug abuse
   i. Uterine anomalies.

Points to Remember

1. Abdominal circumference is most sensitive in 3rd trimester
2. Fetal weight estimation always carries an error of +/- 200 gm
3. Macrosomia is associated with polyhydramnios
4. Shoulder dystocia in labor cannot be predicted
5. Asymmetrical and symmetrical growth restriction can occur together.

5.9 FETAL SURVEILLANCE OR FETAL WELLBEING

When to evaluate:
1. Unexplained fetal death
2. Decreased fetal movements
3. Maternal chronic hypertension
4. Pre-eclampsia (PIH)
5. Maternal diabetes mellitus
6. Chronic renal disease
7. Cyanotic heart disease
8. Rh or other isoimmunization
9. Hemoglobinopathies
10. Immunological disorders
11. Oligohydramnios
12. Polyhydramnios
13. Intrauterine growth retardation
14. Multiple gestations
15. Post-dated pregnancy
16. Preterm labor
17. Premature rupture of membranes
18. History bleeding in first trimester
19. Elderly women
20. ART pregnancies

5.10 BIOPHYSICAL PROFILE (FIG. 5.16)

1. The fetal biophysical profile is a combination of acute and chronic markers
2. The fetal heart rate reactivity (NST), breathing movements, movements and tone are acute markers and are altered by acute hypoxic changes
3. The chronic marker of fetal condition, amniotic fluid is an indicator of chronic fetal distress and is associated with reduction of fetal cardiac output away from non-vital organs.

5.11 EVALUATION BY BIOPHYSICAL PROFILE

1. *Fetal breathing:* Movement is defined as 30 seconds of sustained breathing movement during a 30 minute observation period.

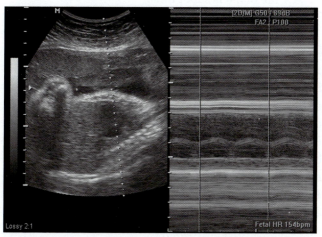

Fig. 5.16: The non-stress test is seen by checking the heart rate before and after fetal movements, to see whether there is any increase for a sufficient period of time or not

2. *Fetal movement:* Three or more gross body movements in a 30 minute observation period

3. *Fetal tone:* One or more episodes of limb motion from a position of flexion to extension and a rapid return to flexion

4. *Fetal reactivity:* Two or more FHR accelerations associated with fetal movement of at least 15 bpm and lasting at least 15 seconds in 20 minutes

5. *Fluid volume:* Presence of a pocket of amniotic fluid that measures at least 1 cm in two perpendicular planes.

5.12 INTERPRETATION OF BIOPHYSICAL PROFILE

Manning score: Each variable is allotted a score of 0-2.

1. A score of > 8 is normal.

2. A score of 6-8 is suboptimal

3. A score of < 6 needs intervention.

The Manning's biophysical profile scoring is a time consuming test (at least 40 minutes). Also it takes into account four acute variables and one chronic variable. Sometimes the acute variables are affected late and remain normal (Score 8/10) while the fetus may be having severe chronic distress (AFI < 5). This makes the Manning's score unpredictable. To avoid this confusion a modified score has been proposed by Vintzelo's which takes only two variables into account.

1. Liquor amnii

2. Fetal NST in response to acoustic stimulation (VAST)

This not only shortens the test duration (less than 20 mins) but also makes interpretation easy and more accurate.

Interpretation

1. AFI < 5. Distress delivery if viable (>28 weeks)
2. If both normal wait for one week
3. *If NST normal but liquor less:* Detailed color Doppler
4. *If liquor normal but NST abnormal:* Acute distress
5. *If both abnormal:* Individualise treatment according to gestational age.

5.13 SERIAL EVALUATION

1. It is recommended that an NST be performed twice a week on all postdated, diabetic, and IUGR patients
2. Patient management is often dictated by the amount of amniotic fluid (postdate and IUGR patients). The detection of fetal anomalies combined with the ability to evaluate the amount of amniotic fluid are frequently stated as advantages of the biophysical profile over additional FHR testing in the form of OCT/CST.

5.14 COLOR DOPPLER

These are done to detect and assess the fetus at risk for death or damage *in utero*. Color Doppler in conjunction with 2D ultrasound and biophysical scoring is now regarded as an indispensable component of a pregnancy sonogram.

5.15 INDICATIONS FOR COLOR DOPPLER

1. Assessment and continued monitoring of the small for gestational age fetus
2. Assessment of the fetus of a mother with systemic lupus erythematous (SLE) and PET

3. Assessment of differing sizes or growth patterns in twins
4. Conjunction with uteroplacental waveforms in the assessment of oligohydramnios.

5.16 INTERPRETATION OF THE WAVEFORMS (FIGS 5.17 TO 5.30)

1. In the absence of an acute incident such as a placental abruption, a small for gestational age fetus with normal umbilical artery waveforms will not develop loss of end-diastolic frequencies within a 7 day period, so that monitoring may be performed weekly
2. Only 10% of fetuses that are demonstrated to be asymmetrically small for gestational age on real-time ultrasound will demonstrate loss of end-diastolic frequencies at any time during their pregnancy
3. Loss of end-diastolic frequencies is associated with an 85% chance that the fetus will be hypoxic *in utero* and a 50% chance that it will also be acidotic
4. The finding of a symmetrically small fetus with absent end-diastolic frequencies in the umbilical artery but with normal uteroplacental waveforms suggest the possibility of a primary fetal cause for the growth retardation such as chromosomal abnormality or a TORCH virus infection
5. Fetuses demonstrating absence of end-diastolic frequencies but which are managed along standard clinical lines have a 40% chance of dying and at least a 25% morbidity rate from necrotizing enterocolitis, hemorrhage or coagulation fracture after birth. The time between loss of end-diastolic frequencies and fetal death appears to differ for each fetus, Following loss of end-diastolic frequencies there are no other

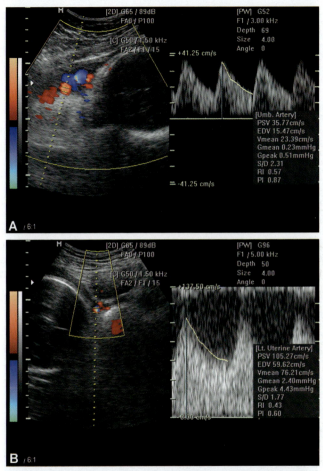

Figs 5.17A and B: Uterine arteries reflect trophoblastic invasion and the prediction of a hypertensive disorder in low-risk mothers and perinatal morbidity and mortality in high-risk mothers. Normal uterine artery flow with flow in diastole and a Resistive Index of less than 0.55 after 22 weeks (Measure the Resistive indices in the (A) right and (B) left uterine arteries)

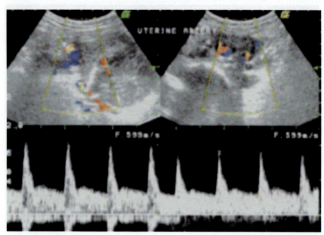

Fig. 5.18: Abnormal waveform showing a notch in early diastole. Other abnormal waveforms can have a systolic notch or a Resistive Index of more than 0.55 or a major right to left variation

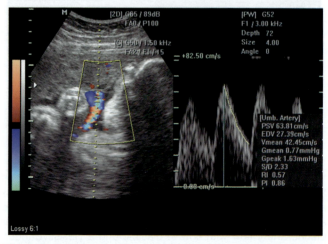

Fig. 5.19: Umbilical arteries reflect placental obliteration and one should have sufficient flow in diastole for a normal waveform

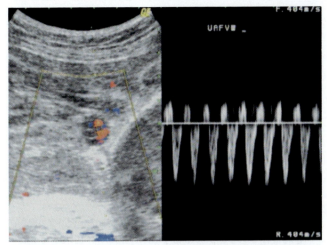

Fig. 5.20: Abnormal waveform has absent end diastolic flow or reversal of end diastolic flow. This waveform shows reversal of flow in diastole

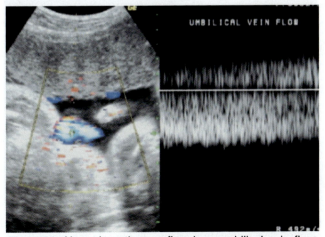

Fig. 5.21: Normal continuous flow in a umbilical vein flow pattern and this reflects myocardial function

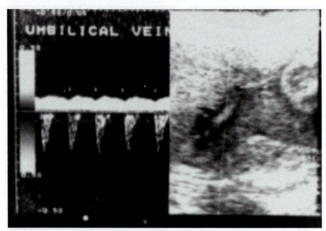

Fig. 5.22: Double pulsatile pattern seen in an abnormal umbilical vein flow pattern

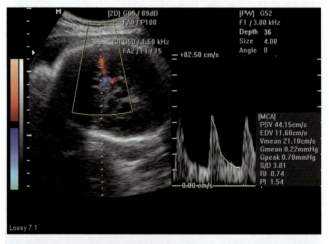

Fig. 5.23: The middle cerebral artery waveform reflects altered cerebral flow or cerebral edema. In hypoxia the blood flow to the middle cerebral artery increases as a reflex redistribution of fetal cardiac output. Normal waveform with a Pulsatility Index of 2.15

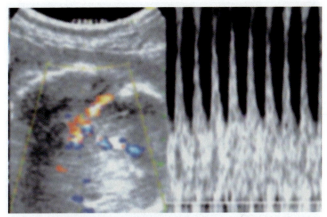

Fig. 5.24: Abnormal waveform with increased blood flow to the middle cerebral artery with a PI of 0.76

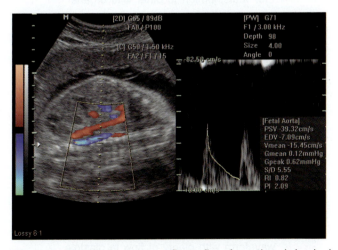

Fig. 5.25: Descending aorta reflects flow from the abdominal viscera and lower limbs. Normal waveform with adequate diastolic flow

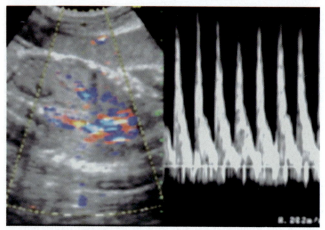

Fig. 5.26: Abnormal waveform with reduced flow in diastole for redistribution to other vital organs

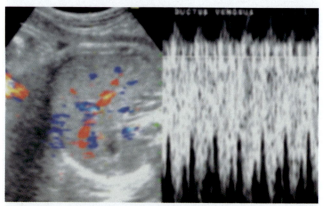

Fig. 5.27: Ductus venosus flow reflects acidosis. Normal waveform with plenty of flow in diastole

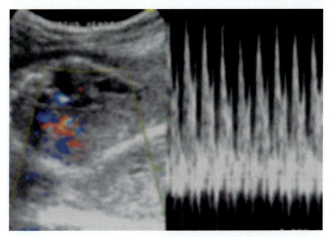

Fig. 5.28: Abnormal waveform with a reduced forward flow in diastole

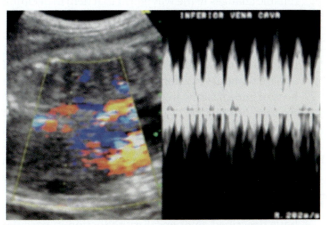

Fig. 5.29: Normal triphasic inferior vena cava flow reflecting myocardial function

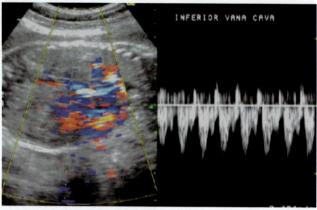

Fig. 5.30: Abnormal waveform with an increased reversed flow in diastole

reliable changes in the waveform that help in deciding when to deliver the baby

6. Reversed frequencies in end-diastolic are only observed in a few fetuses prior to death. This finding is a pre-terminal condition; few if any, fetuses will service without some form of therapeutic intervention

7. Loss of end-diastolic frequencies precedes changes in the cardiotocograph by some 7-42 days in fetuses that have been shown to be small for gestational age on real-time ultrasound. The occurrence of CTG decelerations not related to contractions, together with absent end-diastolic frequencies, carries an extremely poor prognosis

8. In case of IUGR Wladimiroff and colleagues (1986) have described compensatory reduction in vascular resistance in fetal brain during fetal hypoxemia usually called as 'Brain sparing effect' and is the earliest Doppler based marker for IUGR compromised fetus

9. Detection of elevated resistance to flow within fetal descending aorta reflects the decreased vascular resistance associated with high-risk pregnancy not only within the placental vascular bed but also within fetal abdominal viscera
10. Increased resistance in fetal renal arteries with growth retardation has been seen especially with oligohydramnios
11. Increased resistance in uterine artery as indicated by an elevated index of resistance by persistence of an early diastolic notch often precedes the onset of growth retardation
12. The details of normal and abnormal waveforms with their representations and end points and management protocols is discussed in detail in the Step by Step series on Ultrasound and Color Doppler.

5.17 INDICATIONS OF DELIVERY

- Viable fetus AFI < 5
- Absent end-diastolic flow or reversed end-diastolic flow in umbilical artery after 35 weeks
- Abnormal ductus venosus flow > 35 weeks
- Abnormal biophysical profile.

5.18 MODE OF DELIVERY

Vaginal or cesarean section depends on cervical score, pelvis and/or any other obstetric indication for cesarean section.

5.19 ABNORMAL THIRD TRIMESTER

1. Placental aging
2. Separation

3. Oligo/polyhydramnios
4. Cord around neck
5. Thinned lower segment
6. Abnormal presentation
7. IUGR
8. Abnormal biophysical score
9. Abnormal color Doppler studies.

5.20 CHECKLIST

1. Calculate gestation from LMP (keep card with you)
2. Fundal height clinical size
3. Presentation and lie
4. BPD
5. HC
6. AC
7. FL
8. Other limbs
9. High circumference
10. Charts and assess growth.

5.21 DILEMMAS

1. Will the ultrasound tell us the exact date of delivery
2. All parameters give different EDD
3. Has the internal os opened
4. There is a cord around the neck: is it dangerous
5. Has the baby come in the final position
6. How many movements are normal
7. First ultrasound: please check for anomalies
8. Can we wait more.

Index